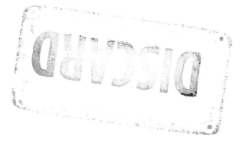

Surgeons and the Scope

Surgeons and the Scope

JAMES R. ZETKA JR.

ILR PRESS *an imprint of*

CORNELL UNIVERSITY PRESS   Ithaca and London

First published 2003 by Cornell University Press

Printed in the United States of America

Library of Congress Cataloging-in-Publication Data

Zetka, James R., 1957–
    Surgeons and the scope / James R. Zetka.
        p. cm. — (Collection on technology and work)
Includes bibliographical references and index.
    ISBN 0-8014-4159-5 (hbk. : alk. paper)
    1. Video endoscopy—Social aspects. 2. Telecommunication in
medicine—Social aspects. 3. Industrial sociology. I. Title. II.
Series.
    RD33.53.Z48 2003
    617′.05—dc21   2003002000

Cornell University Press strives to use environmentally responsible
suppliers and materials to the fullest extent possible in the publishing
of its books. Such materials include vegetable-based, low-VOC inks
and acid-free papers that are recycled, totally chlorine-free, or partly
composed of nonwood fibers. For further information,
visit our website at www.cornellpress.cornell.edu.

Cloth printing   10 9 8 7 6 5 4 3 2 1

Contents

Acknowledgments

Several people contributed to this work. My first and greatest debt is to my wife, Janet Feldgaier, who originally spiked my interest in studying endoscopic laser surgery. Janet's contribution was vital during the interviewing stage of the project. Quite frankly, I probably would have quit without her encouragement and support while I was struggling to hustle up interviews. She was also involved and was extremely helpful in my initial attempts to formulate interpretations and hypotheses from the interview information I elicited from my informants. Without all of Janet's help, this book would be much weaker.

My second debt is to the thirty-seven physicians and surgeons who allowed me to interview them for this project. Without their willingness to teach me about what they did in the operating room with the video and laser technologies, this study would have never gotten off the ground. I learned a great deal about technology and surgical work from my discussions with my informants, and I am very grateful to all of them.

I also thank Howard S. Becker, Richard Lachmann, John Logan, Art Stinchcombe, and John Walsh for useful comments on early drafts of what became chapters 1–3. I especially thank Stephen Barley, the editor of Cornell University Press's series on technology and work, for providing me with unusually detailed and insightful comments and criticisms on the entire manuscript. These comments helped me to improve the book significantly. I would also like to thank Eliot Freidson for his encouraging comments on the final draft of the complete manuscript. Finally, I thank Fran Benson and the staff at Cornell University Press for making the publication process smooth and relatively painless.

Abbreviated early versions of the sections, "Teamwork in Video Laparoscopy" and "Responses to Tight Coupling and Interactive Complexity" in chapter 2, first appeared in the article, "The Technological Foundations of Task-Coordinating Structures in New Work Organizations: Theoretical Notes from the Case of Abdominal Surgery," *Work and Occupations* 25(3): 356–379, 1998. Much abbreviated versions of the sections, "Challenge to Diagnostic Acumen as the Core Medical Virtue" and "From Diagnosticians to Craft Challengers" in chapter 5, "General Surgery Embraces the Scope" in chapter 7, and a brief summary of the overall argument presented in chapter 8, first appeared in the article, "Occupational Divisions of Labor and Their Technology Politics: The Case of Surgical Scopes and Gastrointestinal Medicine," *Social Forces* 79(4): 1495–1520, 2001.

Surgeons and the Scope

Introduction

During the 1980s and 1990s video technology became wedded to a host of endoscopic and laparoscopic approaches in medicine and surgery. This technology enabled physicians to insert miniaturized cameras inside patients' bellies, connect these cameras to television monitors, and view magnified images on screens. By viewing these screen images, physicians could then perform complex operations by snaking instruments to anatomical structures through either a natural orifice (endoscopy) or through small ports punched into the abdominal wall (laparoscopy). Such procedures spared patients from the massive wounds and grueling recoveries associated with conventional surgeries. Demand for these procedures skyrocketed, and the video technology ushered in a surgical revolution.

This revolution is a fascinating case for occupational sociology. The videoscopic technology disrupted workplace routines and, in doing so, threatened surgical skills. This "skill disruption" (see Hodson 1988; Wallace 1989) occurred in an occupation with a secure history of professional dominance (see Freidson 1970a, 1970b, 1986; Starr 1982). How do we explain this unexpected embrace of skill-disrupting technology?

To understand how surgeons responded to the threat and promise of the videoscopic technology, we must first understand how surgeons historically have defined themselves, their work, and their jurisdictional claims in medicine's intraoccupational division of labor. We must determine the new technology's relationship to the core tasks and skills central to surgeons' self-definition and their claims to status and market position (see Zetka and Walsh 1994). As with any occupational group, surgeons historically have been inclined to embrace those innovations that have built upon, and thereby enhanced, their self-defined core skills; they have been inclined to resist those innovations that have threatened these skills (see Van Maanen and Barley 1984, 343–46).

Of course, the actualization of these basic occupational inclinations depends on where surgeons have stood competitively in the larger division of labor within which they cooperate and compete. We must, therefore, map the competitive balance of power in this division of labor. When occupational groups generally adopt disruptive technologies—like the videoscopic technology—they do so primarily as a defense against encroachments on established work jurisdictions. When a group is confronted with the choice of losing control over tasks central to its status position and livelihood or adopting a radical technology, it usually chooses the latter. However, because of its threat to occupational definitions of valued core skills, this choice will not be easy. The new technology may well shake up the occupation's normative order at its core, forcing the occupation to redefine its raison d'être in order to protect its control over the new technology and legitimate its place in the reconstructed occupational order. Surgeons' embrace of the videoscopic technology was no exception to this. *Surgeons and the Scope* documents and explains the occupational outcomes associated with the videoscopic revolution through a "negotiation" framework that sensitizes us to the importance of group-specific, core-skill definitions and competitive occupational dynamics.

Using evidence culled from qualitative interviews (see methodological appendix), chapters 1 and 2 examine in depth the skill demands that the video-laparoscopic technology make upon surgeons and staff in the operating room. Chapter 1 describes the skills that video laparoscopy demands of the directing surgeon and compares and contrasts these skills with those used in conventional surgery. Chapter 2 brings in the surgical team. The types of coordination required among the primary surgeon, the assisting surgeons, and the nursing staff in conventional and laparoscopic surgeries are compared and contrasted. This chapter focuses on what the new technology demands of the interactive system that coordinates operating room tasks.

Taken together, chapters 1 and 2 show that at the behavioral level the new skills demanded by videoscopic surgery are quite different than the skills surgeons had developed and used historically. The video technology shifted the locus of the surgical performance from a direct, tactile environment to an abstract video-screen environment that required different interpretive and hand-eye coordination skills. Although surgical principles and their articulation at the institutional level were not changed fundamentally by this, the basic strategies and routines surgeons used to put these principles into an effective practice were changed. Moreover, the experiential knowledge and skill surgeons had spent years acquiring in open surgery could not be translated easily to the laparoscopic modality. This threatened existing status hierarchies in local surgical markets.

The new technology transformed the nature of teamwork in the operating room as well, as it forced tighter coordination between surgeons and assistants when structures were retracted and dissected. Where primary surgeons, for the most part, controlled the targeted structure unilaterally with two hands in open surgery, four or more hands working instruments from small ports were required in laparoscopy. This demanded an intersubjective form of coordination that was incompatible with surgery's individualistic ethos.

Thus, the new demands of the video-laparoscopic technology connoted a significant skill disruption in surgeons' core work domain—the operating room—and it affected the critical skills required to perform these tasks effectively. This had profound implications for careers and conventional patterns of work organization and control.

The remaining chapters address how and why surgeons embraced this particular skill-disrupting technology. The focus here expands out from the operating room to the larger division of labor, where multiple definitions of skill and occupational virtue coexist. To make this task more manageable, the focus here is exclusively on the specialties of general surgery and gastroenterology. I specify the characteristics of the normative order that enabled each specialty's definition of medical virtue to coexist and function effectively in processing gastrointestinal cases. I then examine how this normative order responded to the challenges and threats of an earlier version of the scope technology—fiber-optic endoscopy—during the 1970s and 1980s. This earlier experience with technological change had a significant impact on general surgeons' responses to video laparoscopy during the 1990s.

Chapter 3 develops the negotiation framework that I use in examining these historical developments. This chapter, the theory chapter, modifies one of the more promising explanatory models in occupational sociology so as to fit the case of the scope technology. Finally, the chapter identifies distinctive features of the medical profession's internal division of labor and sets the stage for the historical analysis that follows.

Chapters 4 and 5 describe how the two major segments of the medical profession's division of labor—internists and surgeons—responded to the promise and threat of the early scope technologies in the early post-World War II period. These early technologies predated the video developments examined in chapters 1 and 2. They did not employ television monitors. Rather, they required physicians to peer directly into the scope from an eyepiece located at the entry port.

Chapter 4, drawing primarily on archival sources, analyzes the cultural frame shaping surgeons' orientation to workplace change with particular reference to their orientation to the early diagnostic scopes. Coming from an occupational culture that lauded efficacy in delivering treatment outcomes as its core skill, and that held a secure and dominant position in the medical profession's internal division of labor, surgeons showed little interest in the early scopes and were content to delegate their development to other specialties.

Chapter 5, again drawing primarily on archival sources, analyzes the cultural frame shaping the gastroenterologists' orientation to the endoscope. The chapter traces the scope's development in gastroenterologists' hands, the conflicts such a development generated(both within the subspecialty itself and the larger intraoccupational division of labor), and the aggressive way in which gastroenterological endoscopists responded to such challenges and conflicts. Both the surgeons' refusal and the gastroenterologists' willingness to embrace the early scopes are understandable in terms of the core-skill definitions each specialty developed from its position in the division of labor. The early development of the endoscope respected the normative order regulating this division of labor and the disparate definitions of occupational skill and virtue coexisting within it.

Chapter 6 steps back and examines the larger institutional and market forces shaping the intraoccupational tensions that were eventually engendered by the development of the scope technology. The chapter specifies the interrelated labor market and institutional forces that undermined surgeons' dominant position in the medical profession and, by doing so, helped shape conflicts over the shift from diagnostic to operative endoscopy, a movement that subsequently challenged surgeons' control over their traditional market turf. Here, we examine federal policies designed to increase the physician labor supply and their impact on the balance of competitive forces within the medical profession's internal division of labor. General surgery responded to state-induced labor market pressures by restricting its labor supply. Gastroenterology, a relatively new subspecialty of internal medicine, saw the state's policies as opportunities for increasing its visibility and status and expanded its numbers accordingly. This created very real market pressures and intensified competition between the specialties. This, in turn, influenced the development of the scope technology.

Chapters 7 and 8 examine the occupational programs general surgeons used to legitimate their attempts to incorporate two scope technologies into their work jurisdiction in response to the increasingly competitive labor market. Chapter 7 examines general surgery's belated embrace of gastrointestinal endoscopy. Chapter 8 examines the history of the video-laparoscopic procedure for gallbladder removal and traces this procedure's rapid diffusion and its consequences. Both chapters discuss the market pressures influencing general surgeons' approaches to these technologies, the programs used to legitimate their hold on them, and the relative degree of success of each program.

The technological experiences documented in chapters 7 and 8 constitute critical comparison cases for theory development. The environmental pressures, the technologies, and the occupational programs examined in each chapter are similar, while the outcomes were different. For the most part, general surgeons' initial attempt to annex operative endoscopy in the 1980s was only marginally successful, while their attempt in the 1990s to establish monopoly closure over procedures that were being shifted from the open-incision to the laparoscopic modality succeeded. In contrasting these similar cases, we can pinpoint critical variables that influenced these divergent outcomes. Here, the relative timing of the specialty's attempt to establish closure around the technology in the course of its development appears to have been important, as was the nature and intensity of the competitive relations existing in the environment at the time of the enclosure attempt.

Finally, chapter 9 discusses the relevance of this case study to our general understanding of technological change in occupational divisions of labor. The case of the incorporation of the videoscopic technology into the surgical craft should sensitize occupational researchers to the general importance of core-skill definitional processes and competitive intraoccupational dynamics to understanding technology politics and outcomes.

1

Skill Disruption in the Surgical Craft

The following example illustrates the basic routine involved in the open procedure used by general surgeons in removing gall-bladders. The basic routine was typical of most major abdominal surgeries performed prior to the advent of operative laparoscopic procedures in the late 1980s.

The Open Gallbladder Case

Sean Mahon arrives at the emergency room of Upstate General Hospital complaining of acute pain in the upper right side of his belly. The surgeon on call suspects gallbladder disease and orders radiological tests that indicate that gallstones are indeed present and the probable source of Mr. Mahon's problems. The surgeon decides that an operation is in order. After some tough talk regarding the consequences of refusing the operation, Mr. Mahon squeamishly consents to gallbladder removal while in the hospital.

Mr. Mahon is prepped and anesthetized in the operating room. The surgeon cuts a deep six-inch incision across the upper right quadrant of Mr. Mahon's abdomen, just below the rib cage. With the aid of an assistant, the surgeon then peels back Mr. Mahon's inner belly layer by layer, cutting through tissue until internal organs are exposed. Moist pads are placed over the wound edges for protection. A retractor is inserted in the wound and opened wide. The stomach is positioned to the left and secured with a pack. Other packs are inserted to protect adjacent structures and to hold them out of the way. The seal between the liver and diaphragm is broken, and two packs are placed behind the liver to drop it and the gallbladder located in its bed below the rib cage for easier access. The positioning and packing secures a workspace large enough for the surgeon's hands to enter deep into the abdominal cavity.

After exposure is secured, the surgeon inspects structures. Clamps are placed on each end of the gallbladder. The surgeon pulls the gallbladder taut with a grasper to expose the membrane lining the liver and small intestine and the point where the separate ducts transporting wastes from the gallbladder and liver join into a single structure. Anatomy here is inflamed and difficult to interpret. The surgeon places the forefinger of her free hand on tissue to distinguish the pulsating arteries supplying each organ from one another and from other tubular structures. All the while the first assistant works closely with the surgeon, holding ancillary structures back to free up access.

After structures are identified, the surgeon dissects and removes the gallbladder from the liver bed. The surgeon pulls on the gallbladder with forceps and runs the forefinger of her free hand between the fluid-filled tissue plane between the gallbladder and liver. The surgeon detaches the gallbladder, using an electrocautery instrument to sever the fibrous strands holding it in place. Once the gallbladder is freed from the liver bed, the surgeon pulls it to the side to better expose the hepatocystic triangle—the point where the cystic duct from the gallbladder and the hepatic duct from the liver converge into a single structure. This structure is dissected out of its bed and examined carefully to assure the surgeon that the duct and artery serving the gallbladder are properly identified. Once she is satisfied that she has identified and clamped the proper structures, the surgeon dissects the cystic duct and artery, freeing the gallbladder completely. The surgeon then inserts an endoscope into the open duct to search for stones. None are found.

After the cystic duct and artery are dissected, the surgeon relaxes. She removes the severed gallbladder from the abdomen and places it on a specimen tray. Then she clears, cleans, and inspects the abdominal cavity. The surgeon declares success. All equipment is identified, packing pads are removed from the abdomen, structures are repositioned. Finally, the assistant sews up the patient's belly layer by layer.

The operation unfolded with considerable speed. Tense moments occurred when the inflamed ductal anatomy was being identified and dissected. The routine involved the assistant pulling structures away while the surgeon worked in the belly, feeling and placing tissue with one hand, clamping and then cutting with small tools held in the other.

In less than two hours Mr. Mahon is resting in the recovery room. He will spend a week in the hospital and then four to six weeks recovering at home before he returns to work. While his belly will be quite sore during recovery, and while he will carry a big scar for life, the painful symptoms that drove him to seek help in the emergency room will never return. The source that produced his gallstones has been incapacitated and removed.[1]

The observer is struck by the low-tech nature of this complicated procedure. The instruments used are all small, hand-held devices. Scalpels and scissors are the primary cutters. The electrocautery instrument used for some dissection and for coagulating bleeding sources is a pen-like device within which an electric current flows. The observer is also struck by how much is done by the surgeon's gloved hands—tissue manipulation, structure identification, even dissection. Although the surgeon made the procedure look easy, its success was contingent upon her well-honed skills. Judgments were made throughout the procedure as anatomy was interpreted and as decisions were made regarding how to manipulate it. This type of procedure and the skills it demands were standard in open abdominal surgeries prior to the advent of video laparoscopy.

Work Skills in Conventional Surgery

Surgery is craft work. Its success cannot be assured by the routinized application of general surgical principles to all cases encountered. Surgeons themselves tend to define their work not as science but as art. Some are thought to have the special calling; others are thought to be incapable of mastering the unique skills required. These skills are thought to be mysterious, indeterminate, and innately held. Indeed, Robert Glaser (1966, 14) reports that a prominent surgeon objected to the merging of the Harvard Medical School with Harvard University in 1869 because, in his view, "surgeons are born, not made, and that the inevitable reduction in numbers might exclude a genius in the art" (see also Bosk 1979, 92; Knafl and Burkett 1975, 399).

Surgery is defined in this occupational culture as an art because of the variable nature of the raw material with which surgeons work. Each patient's anatomy is somewhat different. There is considerable variation as to size, shape, texture, and location of basic structures (ArchS 1994f; see also Fox 1957). Because of this, procedures do not lend themselves to rote standardization. As stated by a young urological surgeon, "anatomy, no matter how you want to cut, slice it, or dice it, it is statistical. One tissue is not the same as another one. . . . So, there is a chance that there is a variation that is significant. There is a tendency to overlook this fact. . . . Anatomy is statistical; it is not tactile. You have to remember those things."

Disease affects tissue differently, making structure identification difficult. Many intra-abdominal formations such as cysts, fibroids, kidney stones, and gallstones do not follow simple patterns, which makes their location and relationships to natural structures variable from case to case and quite difficult to interpret. These can cause serious, unexpected difficulties in the operating room. As an experienced gynecological surgeon put it, "[Take an] ovarian cyst. It doesn't sound like much compared to a quote hysterectomy, which sounds like a big procedure. But the cyst may take three times as much time and be twice as difficult, with higher risk because of the anatomy and the other structures that are involved."

The anatomy in the upper right quadrant of the abdomen is especially difficult to interpret. Many structures are tightly packed there: the liver and gallbladder, the cystic duct and artery serving the gallbladder, the common bile duct, and the hepatic artery serving the liver (AJS 1993c). The gallbladder sits in the liver bed, and normally the arteries supplying both organs look similar, as do the ducts transporting wastes from them. The cystic and common bile ducts actually fuse as they pass down from their respective organs. Anatomy often develops strangely here (AJS 1991n; SCNA 1994b). Studies of cadavers suggest that significant variation occurs in as much as 65 percent of cases. Structures fuse together (ArchS 1994f). Bleeders lie hidden beneath structures in unexpected ways, often behind the duct to be dissected. Because of this, it is easy to confuse the ducts, clamp the wrong structure, hit a bleeder, or injure an organ. Such mistakes can have dire consequences.

Because of the uncertainties involved in working in this environment, surgical principles are useful as heuristic abstractions for guiding action. Success depends on interpretation and judgment in each case. Surgeons must be on guard against an unexpected contingency arising in even their most common surgeries. Developing the type of surgical judgment required for making wise decisions regarding when to operate and how to operate in response to variable contingencies is defined as the most important component of successful surgical work. The traits of a mature surgeon are acknowledging an obdurate, complex, and uncertain environment; adapting one's work routines to manage this environment to the best extent possible; and dealing effectively with the psychological and philosophical ramifications of feeling frequently overwhelmed and of failing to accomplish objectives in a portion of one's trials (see Lancet 1987).

Of course, surgery involves a manual performance, and developing "good hands" for this is very important. Surgeons must use their gloved hands skillfully in assessing and manipulating tissue. Performance skills must be honed through repeated trials (Morris 1935, 117).

Good hands are not only important for manipulating, dissecting, and suturing tissue. Experienced surgeons must learn to trust what their hands tell them and to make judgments during a case performance on the basis of sensory feedback coming through them. As stated by a young colon and rectal surgeon, "When I do an operation for a cancer, I touch things. I like to have feedback. . . . Tactile sensation is really important in medicine. . . . You feel [the colon], and you feel for lymph glands. You are feeling for associated other problems" (see also JAMA 1989b; Morris 1935, 117). A senior general surgeon also said, "If you are doing it open, and you are an excellent surgeon, you have everything in your hands and fingers and you feel. And you develop a certain tactile intelligence."

Because of the importance of feel, large incisions are necessary for positioning surgeons' hands in the body cavity. They enable surgeons to have immediate access to the area they are treating. Such access cuts down the potential for errors. When surgeons can manipulate tissue easily with their hands, and their view of their work object is better, they gain a stronger sense of control over the situation. This enables surgeons to manage problematic contingencies associated with uncertain anatomy, such as bleeding. As stated by a senior general surgeon, "[In an] open procedure it is easier [to control bleeding] because . . . you have your fingers and you can feel. . . . Sometimes bleeding would be of no consequence in the open procedure . . . because of your access and because you can get at the bleeder almost immediately."

Large incisions are also important in surgical diagnosis. The methods employed to diagnose abdominal conditions prior to incision are indirect. Errors are possible and surprisingly frequent. Effective use of the indirect modalities also usually requires that physicians suspect a condition prior to searching for it. Open incisions, on the other hand, put surgeons directly at the site of diseased tissue where they can see and feel it if necessary. As a surgeon stated in commentary, "Sometimes the real nature of the pathologic findings can be appreciated only by holding tissue between the fingers (SCNA 1994a, 741)."

Although necessary in the open surgical modality, large incisions are quite costly to patients. Bellies are cut open, muscles are severed, and organs are repositioned and held back in unnatural positions. To make all of this bearable, patients are anesthetized with drugs that can be lethal. This basic fact affects a surgeon's approach, for it puts a premium on speed and decisiveness. The quicker the surgeon can get in, diagnose, complete the procedure, get out, and sew up, the better the recovery. When the procedure is completed quickly, less anesthesia is pumped into the patient and the patient experiences less trauma. Surgeons are aware of this. They measure their successes in terms of surgical time (see Morris 1935, 154–58, 179–81).

Thus, the video technology was introduced into a work setting dominated by a strong occupational culture that embraced the principles of surgical judgment, good hands, and large incisions. Surgical judgment develops in response to the existential difficulties inherent in working with varied and unpredictable anatomy. It denotes a type of wisdom that is acquired over time through direct experience. This attribute is the core skill that is most highly valued in the surgical culture. Surgical judgment is what separates good surgeons from poor ones. Good hands are the action counterpart to surgical judgment. The concept denotes working wisely in a treatment modality that demands quickness, instantaneous responses to contingencies, and manual dexterity. Large incisions create workspace within which surgeons put their good judgment and their good hands into effective practice. As such, they are critical components of successful surgical work in the open modality.

Laparoscopic Fibroid Case

Dorothy Johnson sees her gynecologist for abnormal menstrual bleeding and an inability to conceive. The gynecologist suspects fibroids—noncancerous tumors that develop in the uterus. After she receives the results of preliminary diagnostic tests, the gynecologist schedules a diagnostic laparoscopy at Upstate Community Hospital and elicits Ms. Johnson's permission to perform the range of operative procedures that are indicated by the examination.

In the operating room, Ms. Johnson is prepped and anesthetized for the procedure as the surgical team scrubs. To begin the procedure, the gynecological surgeon makes a small puncture wound with a scalpel just below Ms. Johnson's navel. She examines the wound by inserting her finger into it and feeling for misplaced bowel or other anomalies. Once the pathway is deemed clear, a hollow, ten-millimeter cylindrical trocar is inserted into the puncture wound and secured. A tube connected to the trocar then pumps in carbon dioxide, blowing up Ms. Johnson's belly. Ms. Johnson is tilted backwards slightly on the operating table. The carbon dioxide filling her abdomen, and the tilting, separate the bowel near the abdominal wall from the internal pelvic structures. This creates a gaseous intra-abdominal workspace for instruments inside Ms. Johnson's closed belly.

To inspect structures, the gynecologist inserts the laparoscope—a long, slender rod with a camera chip on its end—into the trocar. The laparoscope projects an image of the inner abdominal structures onto two television screens, one on each side of the patient's head. The gynecologist stands on the right and watches the left television screen; her surgical assistant stands on the left and watches the right screen. The color image projected onto the monitors is crisp and sharp. A red structure—the patient's uterus—comes into full view. It is large and appears heart-shaped with one lobe grayish white. The grayish-white lobe is the fibroid that is causing Ms. Johnson's problems. The gynecologist moves the laparoscope in the inner abdomen from the handle that protrudes above the trocar outside of the patient's belly. The trocar encasing the laparoscope moves at the base of the port, much like the joysticks used in video games. The gynecologist moves the laparoscope inside the trocar to examine the fibroid, controlling its position from the instrument handle. She decides that she can dissect the fibroid safely.

After the inner abdomen is inspected, the assistant takes control of the laparoscope and holds it steady so as to free the gynecologist's hands for other tasks. The gynecologist takes a smaller trocar and punches it into the abdomen below and to the right of the navel. She pushes the trocar deep into the belly before it punctures an opening. The staff watches television monitors as the flesh indents from the inside and then opens up for the trocar. This port is used for inserting cutting instruments. Two additional trocars are inserted at strategic points in the abdomen and serve as ports for grasping instruments. The assistant takes over the graspers, holding and pulling the fibroid as the surgeon dissects. The assistant coordinates her activities with the gynecologist's, as she begins to cut the fibroid from the uterus.

The gynecologist uses an electrocautery instrument for cutting tissue and for coagulating bleeders. This instrument is a long cylindrical wand with a fork at the end. Electric current flows through the wand and makes contact with tissue at the tines. The surgeon activates the electric current by foot pedal. Holding the camera stationary with her left hand, she operates the cutting instrument with her right. She pushes the fork into the fibroid as the assistant retracts, then she steps on the pedal to zap tissue with electricity, slowly dissecting the fibroid from the uterus in doing so. After a number of applications, the fibroid is detached completely from the uterus. It is then dissected into smaller pieces in the closed abdomen and sucked out piece by piece through the main trocar port. After this is done, the surgeon declares the operation a success. The abdominal cavity is inspected and deflated. The puncture wounds are sewn up with a few stitches each.

The next day the surgeon tells Ms. Johnson that, although she had a large fibroid tumor, she is a lucky woman. Had she experienced her condition just two years earlier, the surgeon would have performed a complete abdominal hysterectomy and would have removed Ms. Johnson's reproductive organs. With the laparoscopic procedure, Ms. Johnson goes home the day after her surgery with her uterus and ovaries intact.[2]

The contrast between the laparoscopic and the open-incision cases is pointed. A strange thing happens when the intra-abdominal image is projected on the television monitors: Reality is inverted. The larger-than-life image projected onto the television screen replaces the patient's body as the focus of attention. This image becomes the real, while the patient's body serves as a mere base from which the surgeon and her assistant manipulate their lever-like instruments. The surgeon did not look directly at the tissue she was working on inside the body. Her hands were not in the picture that was projected onto the screen; they were hovering over the abdomen and guiding instruments that protruded from the puncture ports. Everything was done at a distance. The skills of the gynecologist and her assistant made the entire procedure appear simple, but this appearance belies the operation's complexity. In fact, working from the video screen demands new surgical skills and a different type of action orientation.

Work Skills in Video-Laparoscopic Surgery

Videoscopic surgery is not totally new. In fact, most videoscopic surgeries employ the basic procedures used in open surgeries (see AJS 1991n; SCNA 1994a, 1994c). The theoretical knowledge guiding these procedures is the same. The skill of interpreting anatomy and making judgments regarding how to manipulate it—surgeons' self-defined core skill—also transfers from modality to modality. As stated by an experienced obstetrical-gynecological (ob/gyn) surgeon, "The whole gist of this thing is to do the exact surgery that you do in an open form through a scope. It shouldn't be any different. . . . You shouldn't be thinking any other way." However, knowing what needs to be done and actually doing it through the scope is a different matter. New skills are required for this.

Ecological and Technical Environment

In open procedures direct vision and feel are vital for interpreting and manipulating anatomy. Although vision is the most vital sense used, good hands are a necessary complement to it. Access is always problematic. The space required for positioning hands in the abdominal cavity is difficult to secure. There are limits as to how close surgeons' eyes can get to tissue without contaminating the patient, and tactile sensation and physical manipulation become important to compensate for this limitation.

Spatial dynamics are different in videoscopic surgery. The carbon dioxide pumped into the abdomen separates bowel from the inner structures of interest, thereby creating an empty gaseous space in the closed belly for surgical instruments. Where in open surgery surgeons simply reach in through the opening created by the large incision to access structures, in videoscopic surgery surgeons' access is limited to three or four small ports.

Port placement directly impacts surgeons' access (AJS 1991b). This is especially true for reconstructive procedures or those involving removal of abnormal structures—such as noncancerous tumors—that can develop anywhere in the abdominal cavity. Poor port placement is a common problem with neophytes. As stated by a young ob/gyn surgeon, "That's another common mistake starting out. They don't think before they place their ports. They place them in areas where the area of access to the place they want to work is not ideal."

There can be complications associated with the initial port placement. There are two approaches: one is to punch a sharp trocar blindly into the abdomen. This was done early on to "virgin" bellies (those with no prior surgeries). Although usually safe, the approach can sometimes injure bowel or cause bleeding if the trocar hits an aberrant artery (AJS 1991b, 1993c; JRM 1992b). Because the camera is focused away from the abdominal wall, such injuries can be missed and can cause serious complications. A more conservative approach can prevent this. Here, the surgeon makes a small incision at the navel, manually inspecting the wound for bleeders or for misplaced bowel. Once the pathway is clear, a special trocar is inserted into the wound and secured (GynO 1993; JRM 1992b; SCNA 1994e, 756). Because of the safety factor, this approach was becoming more popular in the 1990s.

Working with long instruments through these small ports can be problematic. The range of motion with these instruments is limited. This makes suturing and intracorporeal tying very difficult (AJS 1993c). One can appreciate this by imagining what it must be like to tie a knot through tissue from a distance with instruments eighteen inches long inserted through ports five to ten millimeters in diameter.

Finally, the small ports hinder a videoscopic surgeon's ability to remove structures. This is not problematic for some procedures, such as anatomical repair where no structures are removed or in the removal of flexible structures. Large structures are difficult to remove, however, and many video surgeons will not attempt to remove them laparoscopically (BJU 1994a; JU 1991a; OG 1993). As stated by an experienced ob/gyn surgeon, "When I do a hysterectomy, and I find that the uterus is big and I'm going to struggle to remove it, I am not going to do that. Because I personally am not convinced that there is an advantage at that stage because patients under laparoscope are under anesthesia longer times than if you went conventional. . . . If you are going to go over three hours, you are putting patients through anesthesia and other risks. So you better quit and go to conventional at that point."

Techniques have been developed for removing larger structures laparoscopically. These involve dissecting them into smaller pieces, holding these pieces in a container inserted through a trocar inside the body cavity, and then passing them through the scope (OG 1993, 471). These procedures require additional equipment and can be time consuming. In gynecological surgery larger structures can be passed through the cervix and removed through an incision at the vagina. In general surgery gallbladder removal was the first procedure that was tackled laparoscopically. The gallbladder is hollow and flexible—ideal for laparoscopic removal. However, even gallbladders can be difficult. As one young general surgeon described it, "Once you get the gallbladder off of the liver . . . we open it, we pull it out through an incision. Once we get the tip out, we can open it and sort of suck out the liquid until it collapses. It is sort of like a big balloon. It collapses. And, if there are big stones, we reach down in there with forceps and start to break up the stones and bring it out. Sometimes the most difficult thing is getting the gallbladder out of the hole."

In addition to ecological limitations, there are some obvious technical ones. Videoscopic surgery is dependent on the workings of several electronic devices—miniaturized cameras, color television monitors, gas insufflators, electrocautery or laser machines. An equipment failure can cause serious headaches. As stated by a senior ob/gyn surgeon, "The bulb will fail on you. For some reason or other no matter what we have set up, we don't get adequate light. We cannot find the source being wrong. Sometimes if you get any bleeding, or if you get some secretions . . . it gets on the scope itself, and it may cause a haze, and you get a fuzzy look on the TV, you know, like you got snow on it. So, there are a whole store of technical reasons. . . . I have encountered times where, no matter what we do . . . it is just not working." Such problems force surgeons to develop a good deal of technical knowledge for use in troubleshooting.

New Videoscopic Skills

INTERPRETING ANATOMY

The opportunity to manipulate tissue manually is diminished in laparoscopic surgery. Surgeons cannot reach into the open abdomen and grab tissue. However, when I suggested in one interview that tactile sensation was lost, the urologist handed me a pair of laparoscopic scissors and asked me to touch his hand with them to demonstrate that through them you could get a sense of feel. Videoscopic surgeons do develop such a sense. As stated by a young ob/gyn surgeon, "You can develop a sense of touch through the instruments as well. I think that that takes a little bit of time. But as your skills increase, you get a sense of that. . . . You can feel resistance. You can feel textures." However, this sensation is different than feel through the glove. As stated by another young ob/gyn surgeon, "You still don't have the same exposure and ability to manipulate tissue and the ability to see or find nooks and crannies with the laparoscope that you could with your hands in the open belly (see also FS 1991; SCNA 1994a)."

To compensate, videoscopic surgeons develop perceptual skills in interpreting anatomy from their television screens. However, the learning curve for developing these skills is quite steep. The screen images are not identical to the direct images surgeons see with binocular vision in open procedures. This has advantages and disadvantages. On the plus side the images are magnified, allowing surgeons to get much closer views of structures and tissues than they could ever get before. As stated by a young ob/gyn surgeon, "You can bring the laparoscope very close to tissue that normally you couldn't bring your eye that close [to] without contaminating the patient. You look at things much more closely and get a magnified sense. You get an idea of what is there, whereas before you couldn't look as closely, and you might have to feel to supplement what you think you are looking at."

On the negative side, the two-dimensional images on the screen distort three-dimensional reality (AJS 1991n; JAMA 1992, 1994; Lancet 1993a; OGS 1993). Because of this, videoscopic surgeons must interpret these images on the basis of their experiential knowledge. This is accomplished with the eye without the aid of touch. As stated by a senior general surgeon, "You are looking at the tissue on the screen. You have to identify it. And, you know what? You have to have an artistic eye. You have to be able to analyze what you are seeing different than if you are doing it open . . . [where] you have everything in your hands and fingers and you feel." This identification process involves a conscious, perhaps subconscious, adjustment. The television image is measured against a mental construct surgeons develop from experience. The type of "artistic eye" required for this does not have a counterpart in open procedures.

Too much faith in the screen image can be dangerous. The view can actually appear better than reality. Clarity and color are exceptionally good with the latest technology. Exposure can appear better, since the camera lens can be rotated at almost 360 degrees from any point in the abdomen. Once surgeons learn to trust these impressive images, they can be lulled into a false sense of security and control, even to the point of making unwise decisions. As a young urological surgeon put it, "There is a perception that it is surrealistic, that you cannot really injure anything because it is so magnified in front of you. . . . That's where all neophyte microscopic and endoscopic surgeons get into trouble. They forget the basics, and they are overwhelmed by the illumination and clarity of view."

The "surrealistic" image can also lead a neophyte to take brash action when something goes amiss. Bleeding is a case in point. On a magnified screen bleeding looks very different than it does in the open procedure. This can cause undo alarm—even panic (BJU 1994b, 267). As stated by a young ob/gyn surgeon, "[It] looks like somebody is hemorrhaging. . . . In point of fact, it is all magnified . . . so what looks like . . .—oh my gosh, a tremendous amount of bleeding—in point in fact may not be. So, you see the bleeding, and all of a sudden you are panicking, because you see this bleeding. Well, you don't have to panic, necessarily. You can, you know, deal with it in good speed."

COORDINATING TOOL USE

Coordinating one's hand movements while watching a television image is very difficult. The instruments are awkward, with long stems that protrude from the puncture port to the surgeons' hands that are working above the closed abdomen. Surgeons' hands work at a distance of about eighteen inches from tissue. Their hands hover over the abdomen, while only the tips of their instruments inside the port are shown on screen. Surgeons cannot see their hands while working, because their eyes are glued to the monitors. The range of motion surgeons have with these instruments is constrained. To move an instrument in the umbilicus port toward the patient's upper right quadrant, for example, the surgeon must pull the instrument from the base of the port down and to the left. The sweep of the instrument's motion depends on its depth in the abdomen.

Given the awkwardness involved in manipulating the instrumentation one can imagine what it is like to guide these hand motions from a magnified image projected on a video screen. This is the most difficult part of the procedure, for it requires an interpretation of what the two-dimensional television image means in three-dimensional space and an ability to coordinate one's working instruments with one's interpretive eye.

The development of the hand-eye coordination required to work effectively in this environment is complicated by a number of factors. First, the television image is inverted. As put by a senior general surgeon, "It is ass-backward. . . . It's like looking in a mirror and trying to put a pin in your collar. The image is backward in the stomach."

Second, spatial distances cannot be captured and projected accurately onto the television image. This has to be compensated for by the surgeons' interpretive processes. As stated by an experienced general surgeon, "It takes some time to learn where the tip of your instrument really is in respect to the structures that you are seeing. It is two-dimensional. You don't get the three-dimensional field. You have to learn to bring the instrument down to where you want to be operating before you open the blades of the scissors or before you try to cauterize something, because you may, in fact, be farther away from it than you think."

Third, the camera's angle and the angle of the instrument working from the access port affect the motion observed on screen. As stated by a senior ob/gyn surgeon, "You have to learn to keep the camera in the proper perspective. [If] the camera starts to tilt a little bit, the picture you get, instead of being in this plane [lifts two flat parallel palms straight up], it is in this plane [tilts palms about 30 degrees]. So, when you are working, you are not working truly straight on. . . .

Your instrumentation is working straight, but your camera is this way [tilted at 30 degrees], so you are getting a diluted image. You think everything is tilted to the right. It isn't. When you want to go and grasp the structure with an instrument—that's straight. So you have to make sure that you are in the right plane."

Fourth, spatial orientation to the camera is dependent on one's position around the table. If, for example, the surgeon moves to work an instrument in another port, the spatial orientation changes again. As a young ob/gyn surgeon described it, "You are looking at a screen and transferring [cognitively] what you are doing with your hands to what's on the screen. . . . You know, it is hard. I mean you don't know where you are. Once you've oriented yourself and have that all worked out . . . now if you move to a different side of the table, everything has just changed again and you have to retrain your brain."

Because of these factors, the hand-eye coordination necessary for manipulating handheld instruments in videoscopic surgery comes only with much practice. This type of hand-eye coordination does not build on the conventional handicraft skills honed in open surgery; it has little relationship to them. Experienced surgeons will not necessarily be able to transfer the manual skills they have spent years developing to video procedures (AJS 1990a; ARCSE 1991, 100–101; FS 1991).

The use of cutters in laparoscopic surgery also requires adjustments. Conventional surgeons work in the open abdomen with their hands, cutting with a blade. They feel pressure from tissue through the blade. Decisions regarding how deep to cut, how much pressure to apply, and how to manipulate the blade are made on the spot. For conventional surgeons, tactile sensation is very important in accomplishing this task. Videoscopic surgeons, in contrast, cut tissue in a closed abdominal environment by manipulating instruments with their hands from a distance. They use both blade instruments—specially designed scissors and scalpels—and instruments employing powerful, remote energy sources—lasers and electrocautery. The mastery of both types of instruments demands cognitive reorientation and the acquisition of new technical knowledge and skill.

The blade instruments used in laparoscopic video surgery are made to do the same types of things as the conventional instruments. However, these tools are long, narrow, and angled into the abdomen through small ports. Mechanical devices, tripped by hand with the pulling of a trigger above the closed abdomen, activate the cutting mechanisms employed in these instruments. Surgeons cannot apply much force when using these instruments, and the design of the instruments attempts to compensate for this. For example, instruments that allow surgeons to rotate the cutters located at their tips have lessened the problem of struggling with angles. As described by a senior ob/gyn surgeon, "They have rotators on them. So, I have a grasper that I can turn 360 degrees. If this is my grasper [right hand grasps left forefinger], I can turn it this way in the angle that I want. Also, scissors can do the same thing. So, if I want to go in and cut something this way, and if I don't have the right angle, I can angle it 45 degrees and now I can clearly see. So, that is where the instrumentation helps you." The development of instruments that clip tubular tissue inside of the closed abdomen has made the task of tying and stitching much easier. As stated by a senior ob/gyn surgeon, "First of all, they just had a loop that could tie around things. Then, they got a suture that can tie the knot inside and outside, and that takes quite a while. But, now they got clips. You just put the clip over the [tissue]. It is better than going into an intricate tie inside the instrument, which is quite difficult to do and quite time consuming."

Instruments, such as the Endo-GIA stapler, manufactured by U.S. Surgical, have also been designed to increase surgical speed by combining tasks. The Endo-GIA stapler clamps, cuts, and coagulates tissue in the same operation (JRM 1993c). As an experienced ob/gyn surgeon noted, "When this is in place properly, what happens is that you close the two drawers of the staplers, fire the stapler to case. It's just like firing a stapler, just hitting a stapler. What it does is lay down two triple rows of staples on each side. It cuts between these two triple rows, so what you have is tissue that has been severed, but at the same time has been controlled for homeostasis."

The skills required to master these types of special-purpose blade tools are closest to those involved in mastering tools in conventional surgery. Their mechanical functions are similar, and they do provide some limited sensory feedback to the surgeons' hands as they manipulate them. The proliferation of such special-purpose tools, however, did require surgeons to invest considerably in keeping up with technological developments and in mastering the particularities of the specific instruments used. The unusual size and shape of these tools, coupled with the hand-eye coordination demand of the video screen, has required surgeons to invest considerable time and effort in mastering their uses.

Remote energy sources—lasers and electrocautery—are also used in cutting instruments in video surgery. They allow video surgeons to treat tissue in hard-to-access abdominal areas with a much more powerful energy source. These energy sources are connected to long instruments. Surgeons typically control the power of the remote energy sources with dials located on the machines; they control their activation on the tissue site through a foot pedal. As they press on the pedal energy flows through the instrument and zaps where it touches.

Unlike the situation with blade cutters, there is little tactile feedback coming from the tissue when a surgeon uses remote energy sources. Control is more problematic, and the potential for catastrophe is increased. As noted by a senior ob/gyn surgeon in reference to laser energy, "You can put that beam on a spot very easily that can go through the tissue you are working on and go right through to something behind it and into the bowel or into the bladder. It can be a potential source of trouble." An experienced general surgeon, in reference to electrocautery, said, "It may jump from what you are cauterizing to an area close by, so you can injure the common duct, the bowel, the duodenum. Using cautery down in that area [the cystic duct region], you may not see it at the time, but you may get an injury; a couple of days latter you may get a perforation." The mastery of these remote energy sources requires surgeons to make a considerable investment in time and effort.

MANAGING BASIC SURGICAL PROBLEMS

Once video surgeons master the interpretive and manual coordination skills required for videoscopic surgery they confront the same basic problems in the operating room that conventional surgeons do. Surgical judgment becomes even more essential, for environmental limitations hinder surgeons' capacities to respond to basic problems. Videoscopic surgeons do not have the luxury of, say, holding a structure and manipulating it for identification or feeling for a pulse to determine if a structure is vascular. They cannot react instantly, grabbing a structure that slips away or placing pressure where needed. Control over the operating field is lessened, and this can be quite stressful. As a senior ob/gyn surgeon said, "There are significant risks associated with a blind—well, I wouldn't say blind—but you are working inside and you can't get at major vessels and things. . . .

[Vision] is limited. It is not so much that your vision is limited, but your ability to react to it is sometimes limited." And an experienced general surgeon said, "I think that there is a bit less control. It feels like there is a bit less control. I don't find it as stressful now than I did originally, but I think that compared with an open gallbladder, I think that there are more uncertainties. And, if you start having troubles, you may have to do something fairly quickly—that gives you an element of stress that I don't feel as much with an open procedure."

Anatomy has been a problem hindering success in laparoscopic procedures. Difficult anatomy, at times, has prevented surgeons from continuing (ArchS 1994f, 698). The inability to identify anatomical structures with confidence can make the potential benefits of the laparoscopic procedure not worth the risks. One senior general surgeon said, "I recently had a lady who had a gastro-resection many years ago, and she was very fat, and she had dense adhesions. And the anatomy was distorted from the previous gastric surgery. We looked at her for a short time [laparoscopically] and then opened her. It just wasn't worth the risk." Another senior general surgeon said, "If I feel that clinically it is an acute gallbladder, I would rather not do it laparoscopically, because then all of the tissues fuse together and you cannot identify the structures. And if you can't, it is stupid for you to proceed with the procedure [in the laparoscopic modality], because you can do some damage."

Tissue that cannot be manipulated with laparoscopic instruments can force surgeons to open the belly as well. A young general surgeon stated about a case where he switched to open surgery, "I had actually the first one in about a year and a half. I had to open it on Monday. It was gangrenous. And you have to be able to retract the gallbladder in a stepladder. . . . And, if you can't grasp the gallbladder with different types of instruments, you can't do the case. That's what happened, it started to fall apart."

Because of spatial constraints, hitting a bleeder was defined as a major problem. My informants felt more comfortable dealing with bleeding in open surgery. Once blood touches the lens on the laparoscope, videoscopic surgeons completely lose their view of the tissue they are manipulating. As stated by a senior general surgeon, "If you cut . . . the artery and you were not able to identify it, that is what they call the 'red out.' Everything just turns red and you have a couple of minutes to open them up and go in there in the hope that you can find that damned artery. Otherwise, the patient goes into shock."

More variables are introduced in decision making during video-scopic surgery. Unlike conventional surgeons, videoscopic surgeons have a choice of either the laparoscopic or the open-incision modality. Because of spatial limitations, the key to success in videoscopic surgery is to do the complicated procedures through an open incision. Videoscopic surgeons should not be forced into dealing with a dangerous contingency through the scope.

Videoscopic surgeons can avoid such contingencies by making a decision to open the belly and perform the surgery in conventional fashion. They can make this decision prior to laparoscopy on the basis of their review of the patient's history and diagnostic results. Or they can make this decision after examining the abdominal cavity during an initial exploratory laparoscopy prior to making additional puncture wounds.

As was evident above, complications can occur during laparoscopy that may force surgeons to switch to an open procedure during video laparoscopy. When these occur, the wise video surgeon opens the belly immediately and proceeds with a conventional surgery (AJS 1993a).

PERSONALITY AND SURGICAL MODALITIES

There is discussion in the medical literature regarding what is called "the surgeon's personality," an action-oriented personality that is bold, aggressive, decisive, self-confident to the point of being egotistical, and obstinate to the point of being belligerent (Wechsler 1976, 108–109, 114–15; see also Carlton 1978, 133; Cassell 1991, chaps. 2 and 3; Nolen 1970, 201–204, 264). To a point, such an orientation is a necessary requirement for success in open surgery. Surgeons work in an unforgiving environment with marked spatial and temporal restrictions. Surgeons are often the last line of defense for a patient—if they fail, the consequences can be catastrophic. Even when these consequences are not life-and-death in nature, the costs of forcing the patient into subsequent surgery are always high. This pushes surgeons to be heroes in the operating room—to do all they possibly can for patients while their bellies are open. This requires a special ego. I suspect the existential experience itself, aided by normative prescriptions transmitted through residency training, shape this ego accordingly.

However, my informants warn that this type of aggressive personality is not suited for video laparoscopy (AJS 1991l; SCNA 1994c). First, the laparoscopic modality is not the last line of defense, since the option of an open incision is always there. Second, environmental limitations require surgeons to be cautious and careful. To be a "hero" in the laparoscopic environment—to push the limits of one's skills and experience—can be hazardous to the patient. This is evidenced in the following exchange I had with a senior ob/gyn surgeon:

> Surgeon: When they first came out with it, there were terrible complications, which I guess you've heard about. . . . Some patients even died from it.
> Zetka: But, it is standard procedure now, isn't it?
> Surgeon: Yes. They've learned. The problem is if you think you are a hero and "I can do anything," and if you don't know your limitations, that's when you get into trouble.

The action orientation required for videoscopic procedures appears to be one of caution, one that allows surgeons to take humble stock of their competencies so that they do not box themselves into dangerous situations (AJS 1990c; 1991j; 1991l; 1993c, 496; SCNA 1994a, 1994c). This orientation is difficult to adopt. As stated in the following commentary:

> Although it is easy enough to say that a surgeon must recognize the limitations of his or her skill and the limits of the laparoscopic access, it takes a great deal of surgical maturity to understand that the decision to convert is not an admission of defeat. This decision is especially difficult for the competitive surgical psyche, accustomed to success, however evanescent, in all his or her operative encounters. (SCNA 1994f, 777–78)

How did the adoption of video-laparoscopic techniques affect surgeons' self-defined core skills? The answer to this question depends on the level of abstraction we choose. At the very abstract level, the videoscopic approach did not change much. Anatomy, of course, did not change nor did the basic goals pursued in most videoscopic surgeries nor did the theoretical knowledge and principles underlying these goals. "Surgical judgment" as a concept abstracted from practical experience and generalized as an attribute or a virtue was not affected much at all by this technological revolution. As a symbol, this abstraction could transfer rather easily from the conventional to the new videoscopic modality. Success in both modalities was thought to depend on the very same surgical judgment. And this type of cognitive abstraction will be important for understanding general surgeons' successful embrace of the video-laparoscopic modality in subsequent chapters (see Abbott 1988).

However, the new technology was quite disruptive when surgeons tried to translate this symbolic abstraction into concrete operating-room behavior day in and day out. The new technology forced conventional surgeons to change their action orientation, to abandon their conventional skills, and to develop new ones. Videoscopic surgeons had to learn to interpret anatomy from an image projected onto a television screen. In addition to the types of judgments made in conventional surgery, videoscopic surgeons had to learn to make the additional decision of whether to proceed with an operation in closed or open form. They were also faced with the possibility of having to open the abdomen in response to the development of difficult contingencies. All of this increased the complexity of the cognitive aspects of their surgical performances.

Other new practical skills were required as well. Rather than working using their direct vision, videoscopic surgeons had to learn to focus their eyes on the video screen while manipulating awkward instruments on the basis of their interpretations. The acquisition of this skill involved a steep and very different learning curve than that involved in acquiring the manual skills employed in traditional surgery. Thus, while videoscopic surgeons did not have to learn surgical principles all over again, they did have to learn new ways of seeing, interpreting, moving, and thinking that constituted a radical break with their past practice (OGS 1993, 383).

The practical costs to surgeons adopting this technology were high, and these should not be underplayed. My informants warned that many surgeons, while facile in open techniques, were incapable of mastering the new skills. As a senior general surgeon said of video laparoscopy, "[It] is a completely different form of surgery. I know many good surgeons who really should not be doing it. They are excellent with the open surgery . . . but I don't think that they can do it." And an experienced ob/gyn surgeon said, "It has been quoted by some of the big guys that 10 percent or so of the surgeons out there will be able to do it, and do it extremely well. Ten percent will be able to do it, and kind of do it and muddle through, but get it done. Eighty percent shouldn't even be going near the stuff. It's not easy. . . . You have to make a tremendous commitment to learn how to do it and get good at it. Some people never do."

The uncertainties of mastering the new technology created a good deal of anxiety for established practitioners. As stated by an experienced general surgeon, "We had four of us in a group [during the training course], and we operated on four pigs. There was one physician from the Midwest that was just shaking—totally nervous. And it was just a pig! I can imagine what would happen to him in the operating room." Such anxiety is understandable, however. For once this "patient-friendly" surgery was introduced into local labor markets, practitioners' livelihoods began to depend on their ability to provide it as an option to their patients.

Finally, the videoscopic technology threatened established status hierarchies in surgical communities. As an ob/gyn surgeon stated in commentary, "The hyped image of a bright, bold, daring, and imaginative young surgeon enthusiastically embracing new technology inevitably promotes a perception that traditional surgical approaches are, if not obsolete, at least old-fashioned. Conversely, experienced surgeons are afraid that what they do know doesn't count for much anymore (AJOG 1993a, 1698)."

The concerns and anxieties regarding the difficulties of learning this radical new technology appear to have been well founded, given the early course of its history in general surgery (see more in chapter 8). In the early years of laparoscopic gallbladder removal, surgical accident rates skyrocketed. In 1992 the *New York Times* reported that from October 1990 to June 1992 seven patients died on the operating table during laparoscopic gallbladder procedures in New York. Some patients bled to death without the operating team realizing that an artery was damaged. An additional 185 patients suffered major complications. At the time of the report, representatives from the New York State (NYS) Health Department told reporters they were receiving weekly notifications of three to four serious complications from the technique (NYT 1992; see also AJS 1993b, 1993f; JAMA 1992; Lancet 1992; SCNA 1994b). These rates were unheard of with the open procedure. Had these mishaps continued they might well have jeopardized the technology's future. Although the causes of these accidents were multiple, the novel skills that the new technology demanded in the operating room were undoubtedly a contributing factor. Yet the number of these accidents did decline as surgeons and hospitals adapted and became more proficient.

Notes

1. The fictional case example is a construction based on interview data and descriptions in AJS 1991g, 1993c and SCNA 1994a.

2. The fictional case example is a construction drawn from interviews and from field notes from two procedures observed by the author. For technical descriptions see AJS 1991g, 1991i and BJU 1994b.

2

Teamwork in Conventional and Video Surgery

So far we have focused on how primary surgeons' operating tasks were affected by the various components of videoscopic technology. In reality, however, surgical work is not an atomized performance but a series of coordinated group activities. The key players are the primary surgeon, who manipulates the target structure and performs the essential cutting; the scrub nurse, who assists the surgeon in the abdominal cavity; and the circulating nurse, who prepares the operating room prior to surgery, monitors equipment during surgery, and serves as a runner for supplies as the need arises. Complex operations require an assistant surgeon and, at times, multiple assistants. These surgical assistants aid the primary surgeon in the abdominal cavity.

Videoscopic surgery dramatically transforms the coordination that must take place among primary surgeons, their surgical assistants, and nurses. Interactive complexity increases considerably in this surgical modality. This, combined with the tight coupling of surgical performances that is characteristic of all major surgeries, creates a potential for catastrophes to occur (see Perrow 1984). This potential can be minimized in videoscopic surgery by developing dedicated work teams and by routinizing their group-based activities.

Theoretical Concepts

To compare and contrast interaction systems, we borrow two concepts that Charles Perrow (1984; 1986, 146–54) uses to analyze "normal accidents" in complex organizations: tight coupling and interactive complexity. Tight coupling refers to the extent to which the unit activities of a social system are closely connected to one another in time. When the activity of one unit instantaneously impacts the activity of the next, the system is more tightly coupled. When unit actions do not have a significant effect on one another, or when there is considerable time lag until the effect occurs, the system is more loosely coupled. The nature of this coupling is important because it has a great impact on the effectiveness of the control structures employed to regulate behavior. Tightly coupled systems, according to Perrow, demand centralized authority. Such an authority structure is required to coordinate the rapid exchanges taking place among system units. Loosely coupled systems, on the other hand, can be coordinated effectively with either centralized or decentralized authority.

Operating-room performances are tightly coupled (Coser 1958; Freidson 1970b, 128–29). At times, seconds can mean the difference between success and failure, even life and death. This links task performances to one another in narrow ranges of time. Scrub nurses act to facilitate the speed of the operation by anticipating surgeons' needs and passing instruments on the spot. This frees surgeons to focus attention and energy on their immediate task. Surgical assistants work to facilitate the primary surgeon's speed as well. They pull back and hold structures out of the way while the surgeon retracts and/or dissects. Although these tasks may be relatively simple, tight coupling makes them vital. They must be performed quickly and in a coordinated context. Each participant's task has an instantaneous impact on everyone else's.

Interactive complexity, Perrow's other concept, relates to the nature of the interactions occurring among system units. When unit actors can perform their tasks independently from one another information can flow linearly between them. Here, actors do not have to monitor one another or communicate while performing; their outputs interact with other units in the system only once, usually as inputs to be further processed by the next unit actor in line.

When multiple units must interact constantly and in complex

ways during task performances, interactive complexity is high. Here, acting units cannot accomplish their tasks without communicating and coordinating with other units involved in the interactive system. Complex interactions such as these demand decentralized authority (Perrow 1986, 146–54). Such a control structure empowers actors directly involved in production to monitor outcomes as they unfold and to negotiate collective responses to unexpected developments on the spot. This is the critical variable in Perrow's scheme.

Perrow argues that tightly coupled systems with high levels of interactive complexity have a propensity to produce "normal" accidents. Such systems generate contradictory demands—demands for both centralized authority, in order to program input flows through the system units effectively, and decentralized authority, in order to enable unit actors to monitor and adjust collectively to contingencies. This contradiction makes such systems difficult to monitor and control. Normal accidents are, by definition, not the result of operator or even technical error. They occur even when the system is functioning as planned.

There are significant differences between the types of systems Perrow analyzes and the surgical team. Perrow's systems, such as nuclear and chemical power plants, are large and complex. They are often dominated by technical units with natural or mechanical interactions. In contrast, the surgical team is a more micro system with a limited number of acting units. Although influenced by the larger environment, such teams are largely uncoupled from its forces when surgery actually takes place in the operating room. Human subjects—subjects who think and will—also coordinate the surgical team's activities. Interactions are intersubjective, and this creates new problems as well as new potential for control.

Teamwork in Conventional Surgery

The interactive system in open surgery is tightly coupled with only moderate levels of complexity. Authority is centralized in the task unit with the primary surgeon in complete charge of the case at hand. The staff and assistant react instantly and unquestioningly to the primary's commands. They facilitate his or her speed and efficacy in the abdominal cavity (Cassell 1991, chap. 2; Coser 1958; Freidson 1970b, 128–30; Katz 1981, 1985).

Nursing functions here are not particularly problematic. Role performances can be carried out efficiently with a minimum of coordination. Open operations use standard general-purpose instruments with which nurses are very familiar. Scrub nurses pass instruments to the surgeon. A scrub nurse may be called upon to manage an instrument holding back a structure. When doing this, the surgeon places the instrument and directs the nurse. Although important, this task can be managed by simply following unilateral directions. Circulating nurses do not scrub for the surgical field. They prep the operating room prior to surgery, serve as runners, and monitor equipment (Nolen 1970, 217). This performance does not require surgeons' constant attention. Negotiations are typically minimal, communications basic.

The role of the surgical assistant is, for the most part, determined by the ecology of open surgery. Intra-abdominal structures have to be moved and held back to create workspaces. In most procedures the assistant holds back nontarget structures to expose the structures of interest to the primary surgeon. The primary then performs surgery on the target structures, retracting with one hand, dissecting with the other.[1] The activities of the primary and assistant are usually distinct. Once exposure is achieved, the primary does not have to focus much on the assistant's tasks. As stated by a young general surgeon, "In an open procedure, the surgeon does the retraction. There is a retractor that is attached to the table that does part of it, but then the surgeon does the retraction and the dissection. The assistant is sort of holding other structures, structures not being operated on, out of the way—the bowels, the stomach. So, he or she is not really involved in the procedure per se. He or she is just kind of keeping an open field. You [the primary surgeon] are the one controlling the whole operative field."

Compared to video laparoscopy, the surgical assistant's role performance is not particularly problematic. The assistant's skill is not that essential to the success of open procedures.[2] As stated by an experienced general surgeon, "The assistant has really a smaller role in an open procedure. I can take someone who has no surgical training and get him to assist me. Just say, 'O.K., put your hand here and pull. Hold this retractor here.' I don't think that the assistant needs to be as knowledgeable with the technique as in the laparoscopic procedure." And a young ob/gyn surgeon confirmed, "In conventional surgery, with very different cases, you can get any kind of partner and be able to do the surgery in reasonable fashion. . . . Much of it is common sense."

The use of self-maintaining retractors enables surgeons to minimize their reliance on assistants. These retractors perform the assistant's function. They are de-skilling and labor displacing. Some informants claimed that, with these retractors, they could operate without an assistant. A senior general surgeon said, "In the open, I have done it with just a nurse. All they have to do is hold the retractor and that's it. But now, actually, we got a retractor that is self-maintained. And I can probably take out the gallbladder alone now."

Because the action unfolds under immediate view, primary surgeons have considerable control over assistants. Assistants work under constant surveillance. Primaries can and do compensate for their assistants' inadequacies by redirecting them or by taking over their tools. One young general surgeon put it this way, "When you are directing somebody to do something [in an open surgery] you can point: 'Do this. Do that.' And you have a little bit of control. You can always stick your hand in there, and you can sort of move them."

Assisting usually can be carried out without much verbal communication or conscious coordination. What communication is required is of a basic nature (Katz 1981, 343). As stated by an experienced ob/gyn surgeon, "There are times when you can do an abdominal hysterectomy and not say two words to your assistant and get through the case in forty-five minutes."

In teaching hospitals residents typically perform as assistants. This role is well suited for training purposes in open surgery. It allows residents to learn through direct visualization and to pick up techniques in a hands-on fashion (see, for example, BMB 1986e, 293–94). Because assisting in the open modality does not demand high levels of skill or prior training, surgeries are not compromised (for criticisms, see CJS 1993b). This practice is effective for getting operations done. It is also cost efficient for transmitting skills from one generation to the next.

In sum, conventional surgical procedures are performed in a team setting with tightly coupled role performances. Mere seconds separate the impact of a given action on the actions that others will perform. Levels of interactive complexity, however, are best defined as moderate. This enables primary surgeons to take firm control over their cases, and their dependence on the skills of their surgical assistants and nurses is minimized. Such a system works reasonably well with centralized, on-the-spot authority (Wilson 1954).[3]

Teamwork in Prevideo Laparoscopy

Although general surgeons typically came to videoscopic surgery with previous experience only in open surgery, this was not the only route. Laparoscopy proper predated the video developments of focus here by about twenty years. Laparoscopy developed initially as a diagnostic tool and was used by both gynecologists and some gastroenterologists to inspect the structures of the inner abdomen.

A common operation that ob/gyn surgeons performed laparoscopically, prior to the advent of video surgery, was the banding of fallopian tubes as a birth control method. This procedure involves a one- or two-hole laparoscopy performed by a single surgeon and a scrub and circulating nurse. Prior to the mid-1980s television monitors were not typically used. The operation generally proceeded as follows: A trocar was inserted into the navel and secured, and carbon dioxide was pumped into the patient's abdomen to establish space in which to work. The surgeon then inserted the laparoscope into the trocar and peered through an eyepiece located at the trocar port to identify the fallopian tubes and the points where they were attached to the ovaries. The surgeon generally worked instruments through an operating channel in the trocar. Electrocautery probes were once used to cut and coagulate the fallopian tubes. Later, an instrument with O-ring clamps at its tip was used. O-rings were positioned over the tube, clamped and secured. If a retractor was needed, an additional trocar port was inserted into the abdomen. The scrub nurse could hold the retractor in this port, after the surgeon placed it while looking directly through the scope.

Compared with open surgery, prevideo laparoscopy used an interactive system with low levels of complexity. Because only one pair of eyes at a time could view what was taking place inside the closed abdomen, the prevideo technology atomized task performances. In prohibiting the staff from actually viewing the procedure easily; those assisting either became mindless objects, who literally had to be placed in position by the directing surgeon, or they had to anticipate blindly what was going on by watching the surgeon's hands manipulating instruments outside the abdomen. This technology minimized assistants' input. They became mere appendages to the surgeon's mind and eye. However, this was not so consequential inasmuch as prevideo laparoscopy was used for diagnosis and for only minor operations. The latter—such as tubal banding—are defined in the specialty literature as "single-eye—single-hand" procedures (AJOG 1993b, 10).

Teamwork in Video Laparoscopy

Soon after the development of the miniaturized camera chip in 1983 surgeons were able to hook television monitors to the laparoscope and coordinate their activities from the screen image. This freed each member of the surgical team from the technological constraints of the older scopes. The most important impact was on assisting. Once the procedure was projected onto the television monitor, assistants could see what was going on inside the body and could perform their tasks more effectively (AJOG 1992, 1072; BJOG 1992b). This enabled surgeons to tackle more complex procedures. Video laparoscopists soon began to devise techniques for removing inner abdominal structures through the scope. This fundamentally changed the interaction system.

Nursing roles in videoscopic surgery are the same as in conventional surgery. Circulating, or "floating," nurses prep the operating room and act as runners locating and preparing instruments as needed. Scrub nurses scrub in with the surgeons and assist them directly. They prepare and pass instruments. They may even hold retractors in place. Although these functions are not new, they become more complicated in videoscopic surgery.

As discussed previously, videoscopic surgery is very dependent on proper equipment functioning. The camera, television monitors, laser and electrocautery equipment—all are complex machines. The responsibility for keeping this machinery running falls on the shoulders of the circulating nurses. They set up equipment and stand by to troubleshoot (BJOG 1992a). As stated by a senior general surgeon, "When something goes wrong, she has got to know how to fix it. What goes wrong? Sometimes the television screen won't focus correctly, the color is not correct; sometimes the suction lines are not working properly, or the irrigation lines are not working properly. It happens sometimes. The CO_2 tanks run out and they've got to be switched in the middle of the procedure."

The demands of the new equipment make the process of setting up the procedure longer and more difficult, as more machinery has to be prepped and tried out prior to surgery. Some informants thought that two floating nurses were needed to perform this role. Some reported that they experienced initial difficulties with their nursing staff's inability to adapt to the demands of the new equipment. As a young ob/gyn surgeon said, "The biggest hang-up is the assisting skills, because the nurses are not comfortable with the equipment. And, if something goes wrong, there is not a dedicated team. They don't know how to troubleshoot very well. They can do basic things, but if anything is out of the ordinary, they get confused."

Some surgeons dealt with these problems by taking unilateral control in setting up their surgical equipment. Others organized for themselves a dedicated crew with which they worked exclusively. As an experienced ob/gyn surgeon put it, "I think it comes down to the surgeon who has to choreograph the whole thing . . . to set it up. And he or she is going to have to run the show. After awhile, if you are lucky enough to have a semi-dedicated team . . . it is like anything else. You get used to it, and it starts becoming less of a hassle."

The types of problems reported by my informants should be expected in the early stages of any complex innovation. They decrease with experience. Several informants did report that their nursing staff's familiarity with the equipment had gotten better over time. One young ob/gyn surgeon said, "It is a learning curve situation. The nurses who are working with the equipment are good at it now. They are highly trained in their field. It sort of smoothes out as you get the routine down." Some informants reported that they were dependent on their nurses' equipment skills. A senior ob/gyn surgeon said, "We have nurses who are involved in the operative scheme with us who are the experts. If we need a new bulb, they can come in and replace the bulb: one, two, three. If you have a coagulating instrument that isn't coagulating for us, it is either the instrument, the line, or the power source. They have to be able to correct those for us. They have the ability and they are specifically trained. . . . Quite frankly, they understand the instrumentation better than we do."

Although important, the circulating nurses' tasks are only loosely coupled to those of others in the operating room. Their tasks are completed before the actual surgery takes place, unless a glitch develops during the procedure.

The scrub nurses prepare the instrument tray and hand tools to surgeons as needed. Good scrub nurses anticipate surgeons' needs, prepare and hand instruments with minimal instructions. Poor ones have difficulty identifying equipment, which causes surgeons to slow down their work. As a young ob/gyn surgeon expressed it, "If they know how to do this kind of surgery it is a pleasure. Unfortunately, because it is new, many of them don't. So, it is very frustrating to have multiple educational experiences for the nurses, because the equipment is different. The procedures are different. And it gets frustrating. . . . You almost always have someone new who doesn't know what you are talking about, or where to find things, or what you will really need next. So, it can get tiring.

"[You are looking at a screen] and asking for something, and they are saying, 'What? A what?' And that gets aggravating, and it wastes time, and it is stressful."

However, once the instruments were learned, some informants suggested that this basic function was easier in videoscopic surgery. Surgeons used fewer instruments in the laparoscopic case and did not suture as much. Because surgeons were not working with their hands directly in the abdominal cavity, they themselves could reach for instruments without contaminating patients.

Auxiliary duties were often added to the scrub nurse's role because of this. Two informants suggested that good scrub nurses could enhance the speed of the operation by holding trocars in place while surgeons changed instruments. As stated by a young ob/gyn surgeon, "If you are changing the instrument, and the nurse knows simply to hold the port in one position, then you can change your instrument in your hand, and the instrument will automatically go to where you are working. Otherwise, you have to pull back the camera, find the tip of your instrument, and bring it back. It saves time and steps with a skilled worker." Some informants reported using scrub nurses to retract. When the surgeon placed the instrument and set it, the nurse then simply held it in place. Some informants, however, allowed nurses to place instruments. One experienced ob/gyn surgeon said, "If you have an experienced team, you don't have to set anything. The nurse or the assistant will get the structure in view and you won't have to—they will do that by themselves. That's when you have the team approach—it is like a symphony. You have a team working together." And a senior ob/gyn surgeon reported, "Sometimes, if I've got something placed just right, they may even—through one of the ports—place an instrument under our guidance. They can do that. They can even change positions. So, they are an integral part of our procedure."

Operating the camera was a task delegated to nurses during gallbladder surgery at some community hospitals where my informants worked (BJOG 1993). This involved guiding the camera inside of the abdomen and then holding it in place. This is done in concert with the actions of the surgeons. As stated by a senior general surgeon, "They have to learn to get close enough so that the magnification works and not to jump around with [it]. And while dissecting, your camera's here [holds imaginary camera], and sometimes the tip of your instruments will exit the field of view of the camera. They have to learn to move the camera. I try to teach them to keep it on the tip of the instrument—over the tip of the instrument—so that it stays in the field."

In sum, the scrub nurse's role in the interactive system depends on what surgeons demand. If they simply prepare and pass instruments, the level of interactive complexity is not particularly high. If, however, scrub nurses are required to be an integral part of the procedure—if they are required to place instruments and to retract or to operate the video camera—interactive complexity increases. Then, scrub nurses must master the same hand-eye coordination that surgeons develop. They must also learn to coordinate their actions with those of the surgeons on a moment-by-moment basis.

Although many routine laparoscopic procedures—such as banding fallopian tubes—are performed with one surgeon and a scrub-tech, procedures involving complex reconstruction or the removal of a structure from the abdomen require two or more surgeons working together. As in open surgeries, surgical assistants hold structures in place during laparoscopic surgery and provide traction when necessary, while the primary surgeon cuts, cauterizes, and removes the targeted structures of interest. When these basic tasks were kept in mind, interviewed surgeons typically responded that nothing changed in their relationship with assisting surgeons. When asked explicitly about the effects of the television screen, however, surgeons reported that the surgical assistant became much more important to the success of their procedures (AJOG 1992, 1072; 1993b; BJOG 1992a; JU 1991b). As stated by an experienced urologist who assisted in gallbladder surgery, "I think that probably in laparoscopy—not neces- sarily laparoscopy—at least for the gallbladder part of it, the role of the assistant is more important than any other procedure. You can't really do it without somebody else doing it with you. It's not like you make an incision and go to the other side and put a suture here and there. You've got to have somebody else to help. It's not going to be that easy without a good assistant."

Again, ecological differences made the job of retraction in ad- vanced video-laparoscopic surgery different than in open surgery. In open surgery, the assistant primarily holds back nontargeted struc- tures to create work space and access to the structures of interest. The more critical interaction occurs intrasubjectively with the sur- geon's eyes viewing the action, one hand pulling taut the structure of interest and the other hand dissecting with an instrument. Sen- sory feedback is transmitted from the surgeon's eyes and hands to his or her brain. The brain then instantly directs and coordinates the hand motions. This action-reaction is intuitive. Staff are not in- volved directly in it, although they act to facilitate it.

The task of holding back the abdomen is unnecessary in video lapa- roscopy, because carbon dioxide separates the abdominal wall from the target structures of interest. However, the task of manipulating the target structure while it is dissected becomes more complex, since it now involves a division of labor and intersubjective coordi- nation. In laparoscopy the primary surgeon gains access through multiple ports: typically, two ports for holding and manipulating the structure; one for the camera; and one for the operating instrument. Because the primary has only two hands, assistants must now work instruments in two ports, coordinating their actions directly on a moment-by-moment basis with the primary, pulling structures taut as the primary dissects. As described by a young ob/gyn surgeon, "You have to hold the tissue at a certain angle, so that the primary surgeon can either cut it or place the instruments over the tissue. So it's important that they are doing it together." And, by an experi- enced general surgeon, "[The assistant's] primary responsibility is to retract the gallbladder and move it one direction or the other to al- low access and adequate exposure. He sort of substitutes for the abil- ity in an open case to move your head to look at one part or the other. He has to show you those parts."

Take the critical task of clamping and dissecting the cystic duct in laparoscopic gallbladder surgery. In an open procedure the primary alone manipulates this structure and dissects it. In the laparoscopic procedure the assistant exposes the cystic duct with graspers through auxiliary ports. The assistant allows the surgeon to distinguish the cystic duct from the common bile duct by pulling on the gallbladder at its base and stretching the point on the "Y" where the ducts converge. A senior general surgeon elaborated, "The more closed that 'Y' is, the more risk you have in getting the wrong structure. For safety sake, the best thing you can do is stretch that and open up that 'Y' as much as possible. . . . [The assistant] sort of uses the abdominal wall as a fulcrum. The instruments are about that long [makes a measure of about eighteen inches with hands]. He takes it against the abdominal wall and pushes it to open up that 'Y' and then sort of pushes the gallbladder up towards the head of the patient. He is stretching it that way, and I am stretching it this way."

The complex coordination taking place between the surgeon's eyes and hands in the open case, a coordination that is controlled intrasubjectively by the surgeon's brain and nervous system must now be reproduced intersubjectively as a communicative act involving two to three people. Four to six hands must be coordinated in tight sequence.

Working from the screen complicates this moment-by-moment coordination. In open procedures primary surgeons are in the open abdomen dictating and monitoring directly what their assistants do for them. If need be, they can correct or redirect their assistants instantly. This gives primaries a sense of control and confidence to work with almost any assistant. In advanced laparoscopic procedures primary surgeons cannot see their assistants' hands because they work outside of the closed abdomen. The television monitor does not show these hand movements either. As discussed in chapter 1, the type of hand-eye coordination required for surgeons to work on their own from the television screen is difficult to master. With four to six hands acting together this coordination demand becomes exponentially greater.

The surgical assistant's role is perhaps the toughest to master. Assistants must become more active participants in surgery. They watch screens and manipulate structures with long instruments through trocars that are punched into the belly at odd angles. Assistants must translate the images they view on the screen to adjust for their peculiar access angles to structures through trocar ports and then manipulate their instruments effectively in concert with surgeons, taking cues from them and responding instantaneously. This is explained in the following exchange I had with a young urologist:

> Zetka: Does doing laparoscopy, or bringing in the video camera, does that change anything?
> Surgeon: Oh, definitely. It changes everything. The assistant has to work in a relationship to the surgeon at right angles. Videowise that can become very tricky, because the camera has only one perspective. . . . It is a lot more complex than you think.
>
> Normally, when you are open, everything is open and you are looking down with your eyes, right? And the perspective is from where you are looking at it. When everything is closed and there is a camera in there, not only is the surgeon not looking at his perspective, the assistant is not looking at his perspective either. They are both relying on where the camera is. . . . But, I set [the camera] up as a surgeon to work at my advantage—no matter what that is—because I am doing most of the tricky work.
>
> The assistant is almost inevitably at a disadvantage, so he is coming in at an angle that is not normal for his perspective. No matter how you cut it, or do it, the assistant has got trouble. . . . They have to learn a different set of skills. Instead of pointing this way, it is not that way, because of the camera direction. They have to modify [their orientation] to the camera.

Working from the video screen increases interactive complexity between the directing and assisting surgeon. Both actors must coordinate their actions together. It is no longer possible for primary surgeons to control these basic interactions unilaterally. Trust in the competency of one's partner to coordinate his or her basic movements effectively becomes essential to the success of the performance. As stated by an experienced ob/gyn surgeon, "With laparoscopic surgery you are limited with space and you cannot tell somebody to hold this, because it is coordination and you are looking at TV. And if the guy doesn't know to move left or right, looking at the TV, you can't teach them instantly. That's experience. It is a reflex."

Unlike in open procedures, assistants have the same view of structures on the screen as their primary surgeons, even though their access angles are different. Because of this, assistants' perspectives and expertise may be called upon to interpret anatomy and to reassure the primary's judgments. In experienced teams, simple, unilateral control gives way to a more communicative and coordinated relationship. As a senior ob/gyn surgeon put it, "The extra pair of eyes, the extra brain that can tell you if you are too deep or too shallow . . . you have another fellow on the other side of the table who can get a better angle at it than you do. In my own personal experience . . . it is always good to have another fellow who knows what the procedure is, is trained as well as you, if not better. You stay out of trouble and you want that. Sometimes, your assistant will see something from a different point of view that will make your procedure perhaps easier, and you are now looking at it from that point of view. So, it is a give-and-take relationship that is very beneficial."

A senior general surgeon replied similarly, "We work together a lot, and we go back and forth. If my assistant doesn't think that I am in the right plane, or if he doesn't think that I got the right structure, I don't cut it or clip it until we come to an agreement."

Thus, the interactive system is transformed by the peculiar spatial limitations discussed above, by the hand-eye coordination demands put on the assistant working off-center from a video image, and by the extra coordination involved in dividing the labor between the retraction of critical structures and their dissection. Interactive complexity increases. In response, surgeons and assistants may establish a more communicative relationship in interpreting anatomy from the screen and in planning courses of action on the spot.

Time is an important and vital element to the success of any surgery. A new complication associated with prolonged laparoscopic surgery is hypothermia. Gases and fluids are constantly pumped into the abdomen during procedures, and, over time, this decreases a patient's body temperature (JRM 1993a; 1993b, 537). The prolonged laparoscopic surgeries that were relatively common during the introductory stages of the technology were looked upon by the surgical community with alarm, as stated in the following gynecological commentary:

> We all are concerned with six- or ten-hour laparoscopic marathons, after which the patients in the recovery room may have adult respiratory distress, fluid and electrolyte disturbance, or core hypothermia as a consequence of gallons of room-temperature irrigants instilled into the pelvis. In such cases the procedure is certainly not preferable to a more controlled laparotomy. (IJF 1992, 267–68)

In general, complex laparoscopic procedures take longer than conventional surgeries. This makes them politically vulnerable to those committed to open techniques. Videoscopic surgeons are pressured to reduce the operating-room time required to complete their procedures for technical—that is, patient safety and reduced complications—and for political reasons. My informants valued working fast so that operating times approached those of open procedures.

As a consequence, the interactive system is very tightly coupled. Each task performed by a given actor impacts that of the other team member very quickly. Many actions—such as the retraction and dissection of the target structure—are done in concert. This, plus the high level of interactive complexity, produces a system that Perrow defines as prone to unavoidable normal accidents (Perrow 1984; 1986, chap.4). Although I did not hear of catastrophes occurring in my informants' operating rooms, it is easy to imagine how they could occur, especially in operations performed by neophytes or by surgeons who were not used to working together. Such catastrophes were real and reported in the media (NYT 1992; see also AJS 1993b, 1993f; JAMA 1992; Lancet 1992). My informants were aware of this potential from gossip , press reports, and journals, if not from direct experience.

Responses to Tight Coupling and Interactive Complexity

How do surgeons reduce the catastrophic potential of this interactive system? According to Perrow (1984; 1986, chap. 4), a structural contradiction bedevils complex organizations that are tightly coupled and interactively complex. On the one hand, tight coupling requires centralized and unilateral decision-making control in order to direct the output flowing quickly through the system. On the other hand, interactive complexity requires a decentralized authority that empowers those working together to monitor processes on the spot, make ad hoc adjustments to contingencies, and instantly negotiate responses to unanticipated events.

Because these contradictory demands are structural, they are difficult to reconcile. For Perrow, the way to avoid potential catastrophe is to change the system. Decoupling units and instituting decentralized authority is one way to go. Another is to maintain centralized authority and to linearize and simplify unit interactions. If these responses are not possible—given the technology or the output—then we either learn to live with the threat of normal accidents or we learn to live without the outputs such systems produce.

Unlike technical systems composed of natural elements interact-

ing in complex ways—such as those found in nuclear power plants—
the system operating in videoscopic surgery primarily contains human elements with learning capabilities. Here, the contradictory
demands of tight coupling and complex interactions are managed by
routinizing complexity.

The typical response surgeons take to manage interactive complexity is to work with the same dedicated partner with whom they
have built up considerable trust. Interpersonal interactions in such
teams, even of a complex nature, become routinized—almost taken
for granted. Communication becomes attenuated, often even non-
verbal, to facilitate quickness and accuracy. A senior general surgeon
stated, "[My partner] has been assisting me on almost every case that
I have done. So, it's just like a dancing partner. You start to understand each other immediately with a little touch or something. And
you say, 'Where's my working instruments,' and he will move it too.
But sometimes I'll say, 'Stay where you are, don't move it. I want to
finish on this side.' He knows exactly what I am talking [about],
sometimes without going in detail."

A senior ob/gyn surgeon said, "[Another doctor] and I assist one
another practically 100 percent of the time. And we have been working together for years. It is one of the symbiotic types of situations.
We can sort of anticipate each other. Know what we are going to do.
Know what our abilities are, and it gets better."

Comfortable interactive rhythms were built up between team-
mates. Such rhythms could be counted on to produce safe and effective results without much conscious effort. These interactive rhythms
were essential for performing operations quickly and safely and for
reacting effectively to contingent problems. As stated by a young ob/
gyn surgeon, "I have the luxury that my [working partner, also a personal relation] is skilled in this. So we basically scrub almost always
together. . . . We operate together frequently and we know each
other's skills, and eventually there becomes a silent communication
among the partners. If you scrub together all the time, you know
what the person is going to do next, and you can do things to make
that task easier for the person. . . . You need someone [like that], because . . . as soon as you start to run into a little bit of a problem, you
can nip it in the bud and it remains a small problem. If you can't nip
it in the bud—as an inexperienced person would not allow you to do
that—all of a sudden you wind up with a bigger problem, a complication where you might have to open the belly."

Surgeons who were used to working habitually with a partner

noted the difference in the length of time the surgery took when they were forced to work with a resident or with someone with whom they were unfamiliar. As a young ob/gyn surgeon put it, "[The] big difference is that whenever [my senior partner] does a case at[our community hospital] with me, we can finish the case much earlier. Whenever he goes to [a teaching hospital] to do the surgery, it's one of the residents assisting, and it takes much longer to complete the case, because they are not used to working together." A senior general surgeon said, "I had a medical student today who had to cover for me. She had seen one [laparoscopic procedure]. It took two hours or something, when I usually finish in sixteen or seventeen minutes."

Teaching centers were not ideally suited to meeting the peculiar coordination demands of the new technology. Informants defined the requirement of taking a resident as a surgical assistant as problematic. As an experienced ob/gyn surgeon expressed it, "Sad thing is, you know, many of these places where they conduct these courses and do all of this [to promote advanced laparoscopy], they have their own O.R. [operating room]. They have their own staff. It is like a team. But, somebody like me. When I go [to a teaching hospital with a case], like I can't demand that team. For this particular laparoscopic surgery to go really well, you need a good assistant, or somebody who is already working with you . . . and, I think that that is a real problem. . . . It's a team. That's the thing. You start getting the real process in an institution where they just do that, and there are no residents. When you don't get different residents, I think it works out great."

One young general surgeon suggested that the problem lay in the awkwardness of directing a neophyte from video screens. He stated, "You have to always be turning around in front of the TV screen. The TV screen is behind you, and the person on the other side of the table looks up at the screen over your shoulder. So, I've got to turn around and point to the screen and show him to do this and do that. I think it [working with residents] makes a little more stress on the surgeon than in the open, because you can't exactly show them what to do. And, if you have to help them along, you are now operating from a different perspective when you are reaching over the table."

For advanced laparoscopic procedures, there appears to be a team component to the learning curve (AJS 1990a; 1990b, 489; 1991o). To become skilled, surgeons and their assistants become like old dancing partners, developing the high level of trust that only comes with experience in working together. This routinizes complex communicative interactions and makes their production an intuitive response, more like a reflex than a deliberative effort.

Two-Handed Anomaly

Whereas most informants talked of the importance of the surgical assistants' skills to the success of advanced laparoscopic procedures, three general surgeons did not define them as being so crucial. Two reported they could perform the operation with just a scrub nurse. One stated that a good assistant was more important in open surgery. Gynecologists mentioned that some practitioners were capable of performing advanced video procedures alone with the scrub nurse. How could this be, given what others were reporting? This became a critical anomaly for this study. When, in the latter stage of interviewing, I happened across surgeons who made such claims I encouraged them to elaborate.

The typical approach to dissection in video laparoscopy was to use the following technique: One of the surgeon's hands held the instrument, and the other braced it for better control. This was thought to be the safest and best technique—the standard across the country. Some gynecologists reported using one hand to hold the camera steady and one hand to operate their cutting instruments. In both cases, the assistant was needed to retract as the surgeon cut, making this process the tightly coordinated two-person task discussed above.

Another technique is possible, however. To avoid dependence on the assistant, the surgeon uses two hands in dissection: one to retract by holding and pulling on the target structure with a grasper, the other to dissect with a cutting instrument. This keeps both processes—retraction and dissection—under the surgeon's unilateral control. The assistant merely holds one end of the structure with a grasper, while the surgeon pulls it for traction with his or her opposite hand. To do away with the assistant completely, the clamp attached to the top of the structure can be held stationary by securing the handle of the instrument that protrudes from the puncture port to the operating table or to surgical drapes. Instrument manufacturers have designed special-purpose clamps for this purpose.[4]

This approach reduces interactive complexity by placing both retraction and dissection under the surgeon's unilateral control. However, this technique requires considerable individual-level dexterity in using both hands effectively. One surgeon defined the technique as impractical. Two saw advantages because it freed them from the possible difficulties that come with an unskilled assistant. A young general surgeon said, "I usually use a one-handed technique. If I have to use two hands, I will. In which case the assistant is handling only one retractor as opposed to two." When I asked what the benefit of that was, he replied, "Well, I have more control . . . doing two parts of the procedure, retracting with one hand and dissecting or manipulating structures with the other hand. It is very important to have proper retraction. That is where most of the mistakes or problems occur."

The two-handed anomaly mentioned here was not the standard approach—team coordination was. And, although a few informants talked it up, it is interesting to note that no one at the time of the interviews had actually converted to doing complex laparoscopic procedures this way on a regular basis. The significance of such accounts probably points more to the difficulties of establishing the team relations required of the technique than anything else.

As discussed in the previous chapter, video surgery made new demands on the motor, perceptual, and cognitive skills of individual surgeons. These demands constituted a skill disruption, at least at the level of practical experience. Experienced abdominal surgeons had a good deal of difficulty making the adjustments required for using this technology effectively. Perhaps the most radical new demand of the videoscopic technology, nonetheless, was the team coordination demand discussed in this chapter. The videoscopic technology appears to have shifted the learning curve from an individual to a more team-based level. And, as we will examine more fully in chapter 4, this innovation was accepted in an occupational culture that had long lauded individualism as a core value.

Notes

1. An exception to this general rule is an operation performed in gynecological surgery—total abdominal hysterectomy. Here, assistant surgeons typically perform half of the surgery. If they are positioned at the left side of the table, they will dissect the structures from the abdomen on that side, while the primary surgeon will

dissect the structures on the other side. Again, this is determined by ecology. The ovaries lie on either side of the uterus and are attached to it by the fallopian tubes. A surgeon standing on one side of the table will have difficulties reaching over and working on the opposite side of the abdomen. That ob/gyn surgeons can each do a separate side on their own, and speed up the procedure considerably in doing so, suggests that the level of coupling is not as tight here as in other procedures.

2. This is reflected in Charles Bosk's (1979, 222) assertion that retractors, the fundamental tool employed by the assistant, are known as "idiotsticks" in the surgical culture.

3. For general discussion of authority types with tight coupling, see Perrow (1986, 146–54). William Nolen (1970, 217, 225, 246) mentions that some great surgeons make poor assistants because they refuse to follow orders and are difficult to control.

4. Relatedly, a one-puncture technique was reported in the gynecological literature for laparoscopically assisted hysterectomy (JRM 1992a).

3

Dominance, Competition, and Negotiation within Occupational Divisions of Labor

Chapters 1 and 2 focused attention on how the videoscopic technology affected surgeons' work practices and skills. However, my goal is not simply to describe these outcomes but to explain why they occurred. How do we explain the advent and diffusion of this skill-disruptive technology in a craft-based occupational group with professional dominance over its work process? Why, among alternative possibilities, did this particular development unfold? To answer these questions, we must extend the range of our examination outward from immediate developments in the operating room to the internal division of labor governing competitive relationships in the medical profession. Surgeons did not develop their technological choices in isolation from other medical specialists with whom they cooperated and competed, nor did they develop these choices in a historical vacuum. Rather, I argue that dynamics unleashed from within the medical profession's internal division of labor from the 1960s through the 1980s greatly influenced videoscopic technology's developmental course in general surgery during the 1990s. The remaining chapters of this book document these historical effects.

The Negotiation Model

Since 1980, scholars have increasingly recognized that occupational developments occur within relationship structures, and characteristics of these inter- or intraoccupational structures play an important role in determining how developments unfold (see, for example, Abbott 1988). Although many perspectives contain this insight, one of the more promising recognizes the role that both domination and negotiation plays in establishing turf jurisdictions between potential competitors in occupational divisions of labor. This perspective draws insights from both the Weberian conflict and symbolic interactionist traditions. I refer to it as simply the negotiation perspective. Although a diverse array of studies, guided by diverse perspectives, have used the imagery described below, for simplicity and clarity I gloss their particular differences.

The negotiation perspective embraces Everett Hughes's (1971) recognition of both the complexity of the bundle of tasks performed in the workplace by a given occupational group and the tendency of that group to differentially value these tasks. As discussed in the introduction above, most occupational groups define certain tasks they perform as core tasks central to their sense of self-worth and status. They define other tasks as much less central, and still others as demeaning. Occupational groups care most about their core tasks. They generally attempt to control these performances and establish protective boundaries around them. They define their core task domains as being governed by an indeterminate knowledge base reflecting their unique skills, a type of knowledge base that does not lend itself to routinization (see Jamous and Peloille 1970; see also Baer 1986, 139–41; Boreham 1983, 129–30; Becker et al. 1961; Freidson 1970b, 1994).

However, as Glenn Gritzer (1982) and Gerald Larkin (1983) argue, this drive to control one's task environment and to erect exclusionary boundaries around it does not extend to other tasks. Powerful and dominant occupational groups mold their divisions of labor to protect their control over their self-defined core tasks (see Jamous and Peloille 1970; Walsh 1989). They are largely indifferent as to who controls or performs related work activities, so long as they get done. This leaves considerable room in the division of labor for less powerful occupational groups to compete for leftover tasks, to carve out their own task domains and define the core skills associated with them, and to negotiate autonomy and limited control over these domains with the more powerful groups. The negotiation perspective, thus, recognizes that powerful occupational groups often dominate divisions of labor. It also recognizes that when other occupational groups acknowledge and accept this dominance as legitimate, they can often negotiate outcomes consistent with their own interests and desires. Rue Bucher and her associates have developed conceptual imagery to capture the stages involved in these types of occupational level mobilizations and negotiations (Bucher 1962, 1988; Bucher and Strauss 1961; Strauss et al., 1964; see also Child and Fulk 1982).

Those influenced by the negotiation perspective have specified a typical pattern regarding the embrace of radical technological innovations in occupational divisions of labor. Occupational members generally holding lower status positions first organize new specialties and advance normative claims for control over the new technology. They negotiate with the more powerful segments in the division of labor for task jurisdiction over the new technology's applications and over the new market turf that it makes available (see Bucher 1988).

The established occupational groups in the division of labor often support these jurisdictional claims for a number of reasons. First, the newly specializing groups typically organize to claim turf that is peripheral to that controlled by the more established and powerful groups. Doing so avoids conflict over the more secure markets that the established segments covet and claim. Second, the newly specializing groups agree to shoulder the full costs of adapting to the often-strenuous demands of new technology. The dominant segments are insulated from these costs. Their own core work domains are not affected at all by the demands of the new technology. Third, the new specializing groups' mastery over new technology, and their eventual monopoly closure over the new markets it opens up, gives the larger occupation an advantage over its competitors in the societal division of labor. It enables the larger occupation to expand its jurisdiction and visibility and to increase the legitimacy of its general claim to market turf and status. Under these conditions, such movements create win-win situations for both the dominant and newly mobilizing occupational groups.

The negotiation model sketched above represents an advance over competing theoretical frameworks and has generated important research on occupational dynamics (see Arney 1982; Bucher 1988; Gritzer 1982; Gritzer and Arluke 1985; Halpern 1992; Larkin 1983; Schneller 1978). The model sensitizes us to competing interests in occupational divisions of labor, to the importance of power in influencing developments, and to the complex negotiations that take place between those advancing a program to control a work domain and those with vested interests in securing stability and dominance in the larger division of labor. All of these factors must be accounted for when explaining fully the impact of new technology on work and occupational outcomes.

Unfortunately, the work outcomes of the videoscopic technology under discussion here, on first appearance, seem to be an anomaly to those developments predicted and explained by the negotiation perspective. Although videoscopic technology did hold skill-disrupting potential, it did not produce a separate specialization movement. General surgeons embraced this technology even when it challenged time-honored skills and initially threatened havoc in the operating room. They did not delegate this development in the face of these threats. General surgeons themselves paid the considerable costs involved in adding the videoscopic procedures to their task bundles and in adapting to their demands.

However, the anomaly should not be dismissed or ignored. As we shift our focus from the immediate workplace to the larger historical stage upon which developments unfolded, it will become apparent that general surgeons' ultimate embrace of this skill-disrupting technology was actually a defensive reaction to an earlier development. This development involved attempts to integrate an earlier scope technology—fiber-optic endoscopy—into gastrointestinal medicine's internal division of labor on surgeons' own terms. Surgeons' initial responses to this technology actually followed those depicted in the negotiation model. The technology was, for the most part, delegated to a weaker and lower-status specialty—gastroenterology—and an attempt was made to integrate it into the division of labor in a manner that respected occupational jurisdictions and the competitive balance of forces existing there. However, the normative regulations operating in gastrointestinal medicine's internal division of labor failed to accomplish this integration, the technology ultimately disrupted these time-honored jurisdictional patterns, and the end result was an intensifying turf war. Surgeons embraced the laparoscopic technology in the wake of this normative breakdown, largely as a defensive strategy to secure control over their remaining market turf. Because of this, the case of the videoscopic revolution in general surgery, as understood in its historical context, can serve as a critical case for further theoretical development.

Before we begin to examine the historical case more intensively, an initial refinement is in order. The negotiation perspective requires a more nuanced conceptualization of occupational divisions of labor before we can extend it to cases like that of videoscopic surgery and fiber-optic endoscopy. Occupational divisions of labor typically are portrayed in the negotiation perspective as developing along a segmented course with the activities of each occupational group being loosely coupled to that of others. Once jurisdiction is granted to the occupational group that claims a new technology, the specialty serves its market in relative isolation from other groups in the division of labor. The problem of coordination between specialized groups after initial mobilization is not addressed as problematic and, to the extent that the division of labor in question mirrors this segmented and loosely coupled imagery, it probably isn't. Take the legal profession, for example. If clients are charged with criminal offenses, they consult with a criminal defense lawyer. If they need tax advice, they consult a tax lawyer. Here, there is little need for the legal professionals providing these services to coordinate their work activities with one another. Most occupational divisions of labor probably take this more segmented form.

Another type exists, however. Indeed, an often overlooked, but fundamental, axis of differentiation found in medicine's own internal division of labor is functional rather than segmental. In major medical areas, such as in cardiovascular, neurological, and gastrointestinal medicine, at least two specialties—one from internal medicine, one from surgery—share the same anatomical turf. These specialties provide separate but overlapping services in each of the areas in which they coexist, and they must coordinate their activities accordingly. We must understand this type of functional division of labor, and how its occupational groups coordinate work tasks with one another, to understand the peculiar outcomes of the videoscopic technology. Here, we describe the basic characteristics of this functional division of labor and how occupational groups working within it typically manage its coordination dilemmas.

The Functional Division of Labor in U.S. Medicine

A cursory glimpse suggests little rationality to the division of labor governing the medical profession. Medical specialties have organized around population groups, technology, organ systems, and disease types (see Stevens 1971, 145, 214–16). However, there are

TABLE 1
Approved Medical Residencies in 1970 by Specialty Type

Specialty	Number
Hospital Service	
Pathology	3,727
Radiology	3,136
Anesthesiology	2,099
Total	8,962
Preventative, Rehabilitation, and Occupational based	
Physical medicine	508
Public health	305
aviation medicine	115
occupational medicine	86
Total	1,014
Internist	
Internal medicine	7,970
Pediatrics	2,929
General practice	980
Neurology	914
Dermatology	577
Allergy	99
Surgical	
General Surgery	7,654
Obstetrics and Gynecology	3,070
Orthopedic Surgery	2,102
Opthalmologic Surgery	1,354
Otolaryngology	1,008
Urology	1,001
Neurological Surgery	564
Plastic Surgery	245
Thoracic Surgery	245
Proctology	32
Total	17,275
Total Medical Residencies	40,720

Source: Constructed from information provided in Rosemary Stevens, *American Medicine and the Public Interest* (New Haven: Yale University Press, 1971), 395, table 9.

governing logics at play. As table 1 suggests, there are two primary axes of differentiation: a functional axis that distinguishes specialties associated with internal medicine from surgery; and a segmental axis that distinguishes specialists affiliated with either internal medicine or surgery by anatomy or organ system. With noted exceptions—for example, the important hospital-based specialties of radiology, anesthesiology, and pathology—most medical specialties trace their lineage to either internal medicine or surgery. Most of

these participate in a functional division of labor with sister specialties from the other field. For example, cardiologists and cardiac
surgeons, neurologists and neurosurgeons, rheumatologists and or-
thopedic surgeons, and gastroenterologists and both general and
colon and rectal surgeons all share anatomical turf with the other
party in their respective specialization, even when their training and
worldviews are quite different.

Competing Definitions of Occupational Virtue

The earliest division in the modern medical profession was between medicine and surgery. Prior to the late nineteenth century each
segment had distinctive histories, training institutions, clienteles,
and class origins. Although medical internists do treat patients, they
tend to define the accurate diagnosis of patients' conditions as their
core skill. The application of treatment regimens, whether it takes
the form of swallowing pills, giving injections, or performing anatomical interventions, is not usually defined as having the same status in
the internists' meaning frame. Indeed, internists often delegate such
treatments to patients themselves, to subordinates within the medical team, or to treatment-oriented specialists. From the internists'
viewpoint, the core medical skill, whose mastery demands years of
training and experience, is the cognitive understanding of disease
processes and their case manifestations. The diagnostic skill involved
in eliciting relevant information and in interpreting this information
correctly within the occupation's abstract classification system is defined by them as the most virtuous and essential clinical skill in the
art of medicine (see Atkinson, Reid, and Sheldrake 1977, 258; for general discussion, see Abbott 1988, chap. 2).

To surgeons, on the other hand, "curing" pathological conditions
is the most virtuous skill in the medical arts. Diagnosing the true
pathology of the condition is, in and of itself, irrelevant if doing so
does not lead directly to the improvement of the patient's condition.
Holding this view, surgeons have concentrated their efforts on those
conditions that could be treated successfully through anatomical reconstruction. They have been quick to delegate both diagnostic tasks
and other medical treatments to other physicians.

This distinction between medical and surgical definitional frames
has been accepted, inculcated, and perpetuated in the profession's
training institutions (see Atkinson 1971, 77; Kendall 1963; Nolen

1970, 202–205; see also AJS 1973). Internists and surgeons train together only in the early years of medical school. Once they enter residency training, they part company and are socialized into their chosen specialty's meaning frame. Medical specialties typically train their practitioners in fellowship programs only after they have completed years of postgraduate training in internal medicine. Medical subspecialists are forced to become internists before they become either cardiologists, gastroenterologists, rheumatologists, and the like (AJS 1991a; ArchS 1987; Gas 1979d). Although surgery's hold on its related specialties has been weaker historically, most surgical specialties require at least some training in general surgery, typically one to two years of basic training.[1]

The occupational identification of physicians has also tended to become specialized as a result of these post-M.D. training regimens. Membership in the American Medical Association (AMA) has declined since the 1960s (see Berlant 1975, 183; Feldstein 1977, 27). Membership in specialty associations, in contrast, has risen. Observers have noted that the intense socialization experiences from which physicians develop their occupational identities and worldviews occur in postgraduate training. In describing specialty training at a university hospital internship program in the 1960s, Emily Mumford (1970, 134) writes:

> Experience in the specialty group at University Hospital resembles the time aspects as well as the interaction potential in training of military personnel and training for some religious orders, where individuals seem disposed over time to turn increasingly toward a single professional reference group. . . . Adult training is standardized, prolonged, and intense. In each, the recruit is subject to a highly structured environment almost around the clock; outside contacts are limited, whether by formal regulations or by time demands. Such environments appear capable at times of producing individuals of similar attitudes and behavior, and sometimes even physical bearing. (See also Atkinson 1971; 1981, 113; Becker et al. 1961, 409–10; Bosk 1979; Bucher and Stelling 1977, 661; Carlton 1978; Fox 1989, 109, 125; Kendall 1963)[2]

Coordination and Control in Functional Divisions of Labor

The potential for intraoccupational strife is a serious one, not only for gastrointestinal medicine, but for all occupational divisions of la-

bor. Such divisions of labor decentralize decision-making authority
and task coordination. Work processes are collaborative. Workers in
these systems must themselves be inclined to put aside their narrow
self-interests and "do the right thing" for the sake of the client and
the occupational community.

This normative and communitarian action orientation is generally
inculcated in strong occupations through intensive socialization.
Workers develop distinctive work-centered identities and value systems and become committed and involved members of moral communities, internalizing their standards and practice. The collective
understandings that make up the occupational lore of these communities ultimately guide workers' decisions so that they are consistent with the occupation's ultimate ends (see Hughes 1971, 332–
33; Simpson 1985; Stinchcombe 1959; Trice 1993; Van Maanen and
Barley 1984; on surgeons, see Bosk 1979). The effective functioning
of the nonhierarchical mode of coordination found in occupational
divisions of labor depends upon the generation of these shared understandings (see Barley 1996; Freidson 2001; Stinchcombe 1959; Van
Maanen and Barley 1984).

The problem with medicine's functional division of labor is that
there are dual moral communities competing for the same turf, and
their worldviews and value systems are distinct and potentially competing. This creates much greater potential for dissension and conflict than in more segmented divisions of labor, and this dissention
and conflict cannot be resolved solely through socialization and apprenticeship training. Whose community standards will prevail in
treating a particular case when differences of opinion arise? How
does the division of labor coordinate case flows so that clients see the
appropriate specialists, especially when opinions and protocols dif-
fer between specialties?

These coordination issues are especially problematic for the medical profession's functional division of labor, since the surgical specialties typically delegate the initial diagnosis of the case to others.
Grace De Santis (1980, 214) has suggested that a medical specialty's
structural location in the service delivery work flow—what labor
sociologists refer to as "positional power"—will influence its market orientation. Those in gatekeeping positions with a direct relationship with their clients are more likely to be client or market
responsive. They control directly clients' entrée to the profession's
service delivery system and are not dependent on other segments.

Their level of positional power is therefore quite high. Such gate-keeping segments, according to De Santis, are less influenced by the professional audiences and often do not feel compelled to seek out their support or sanction when engaging in opportunistic market behavior. Those that practice downstream from the gatekeeping positions are dependent upon referrals, their positional power is lower, and they are less inclined toward market opportunism. Our concern here is with how these types of structurally generated power imbalances become regulated so that relative order and efficiency prevails.

I argue that a normative order emerged in the medical profession with internists and surgeons establishing a jurisdictional balance between their respective turfs. Workable scripts emerged for processing cases and preserving this balance. Surgeons established closure over what became defined as the "surgical" cases—those that could be treated more effectively with open surgery—while general practitioners, internists, or other medical specialties processed the "medical" or nonsurgical cases.

Once such definitions became established as hard boundaries, physicians working in gatekeeping positions used them to direct cases to appropriate specialists. Upon initial diagnosis, primary care physicians labeled gastrointestinal symptoms as either medical or surgical. They treated the bulk of the medical cases themselves and referred the much smaller number of surgical cases to the surgeons. If a case defied easy diagnosis, or if it did not get better after the front-line treatment, it went to the gastroenterologist, who would then diagnose the case and, depending on the diagnosis, send it for treatment either back to the primary physician or to the surgeon. As long as these scripts worked reasonably well, specialties with very different training, worldviews, and action orientations could coexist in relative peace and coordinate their work serving the same anatomical turf. Power imbalances between the specialties were kept in check by the normative hold these scripts had over the relevant parties. This normatively regulated, functional division of labor was in place and was working reasonably well in gastrointestinal medicine when fiber-optic endoscopy came on the scene in the 1960s.

In the chapters that follow I document how this division of labor responded to the promise and threat of fiber-optic endoscopy, and how this earlier technological experience influenced surgeons' ultimate embrace of video laparoscopy during the 1990s.

Notes

1. The noted exceptions in abdominal surgery are urology and obstetrics and gynecology. These specialties, perhaps because of their exceptional characteristics, were pioneers in the scope techniques of interest here.

2. Bosk argues (1979, 21, 184–85, 189–90) against Eliot Freidson's portrayal of collegial controls in medicine as being permissive. He holds that the internalization of core values during this critical socialization period is the key component of medicine's control system.

4

General Surgeons' Response to the Early Scopes

Scholars have viewed negatively craft workers' prospects for occupational control. Workers who define their occupational identities on the basis of their manual, performance-based skills are thought to lack the cognitive orientation necessary for responding effectively to technological change. Craft workers do not generalize their experiential skills to an abstract level and, failing to do so, are not in position to make convincing claims for controlling and monopolizing innovative techniques (see Abbott 1988). Because of this, craft workers are depicted as reactionary, stubbornly clinging to outmoded techniques as the march of science, progress, and reason passes them by. Yet by the early decades of the twentieth century the dominant position in U.S. medicine was held not by internists holding the cognitive orientation thought to convey significant status advantages but by surgical craft workers.

Structural Impediments to Dominance

The surgeons' dominant position is remarkable given the early development of the craft, surgeons' downstream position in health care, and patients' reluctance to submit to the knife. First, few medical treatments of any kind were effective prior to the middle of the nineteenth century (ArchS 1989c). Unlike most medical treatments, however, surgery often killed. Without effective anesthetics, abdominal surgeons were forced to work frantically and often sloppily in the open wound before the patient went into shock (AnnS 1985, 423; CJS 1992, 536). And, without adequate understanding of infection, as many as 80 percent of surgical patients suffered gangrene, about half died after major operations. Because of this, open abdominal surgery was not acceptable as an elective procedure. It was a last resort for those facing agonizing death without it (AnnS 1985, 423). With such results, surgeons had difficulty establishing a secure position in medicine.

Second, surgeons held, and continue to hold, a downstream position in health care delivery. Surgeons are structurally dependent on other medical gatekeepers for patient access. This tends to isolate surgeons from their nonsurgical colleagues and keeps them distant from medical advances (AJS 1965c, 119).[1] Medical internists, working upstream, are in position to relegate surgeons to a technician's role in patient care, referring patients to them as a last resort for specific treatments that they deem necessary. Often dependent upon such referrals for their livelihood, some surgeons consent to this restricted role (ArchS 1978a). It is quite difficult to establish a dominant position in such a situation. To win success, the aspiring segment must persuade the upstream segments in their profession of the efficacy of their occupational program. If such segments are not persuaded, or if they feel threatened, the segment struggling to win dominance does not have the resources in the downstream position to force the issue.

Third, patients generally are quite adverse to surgical treatment. The very thought of undergoing major surgery, in the past and now, generates white-knuckled fear. Patients opt for medical treatments even when their outcomes are far inferior to surgery's, even when the surgical risks associated with the needed procedure are relatively slight. No one is more aware of this than surgeons. One surgical commentary states, "An operation is an assault on a fellow human being—legalized, but nonetheless an assault. . . . Faced with a surgical illness, both pauper and president regard us with a mixture of trust, fear, and awe. Their helplessness and dependence at such times may bring with them great gratitude, or, on occasion, great resentment (Surg 1978a, 296; see also SCNA 1982e, 600–601)."

Despite confronting all of these obstacles, surgeons managed to rise to a dominant position in U.S. medicine by the early decades of the twentieth century. Surgeons won this success by delivering the quantifiable treatment outcomes needed for the larger medical profession to secure its general jurisdiction in society.[2] Medicine, even with its arrogant history of defining surgeons as mere craft workers, and even with its attempts to relegate surgery to an inferior status within the occupational division of labor, was forced to embrace surgery's successes as its own and, in doing so, to legitimate surgeons' claims to a dominant position.

Surgery's Ascendance

Historically, surgery's position in the medical division of labor has been uncertain and precarious. In Britain, medicine and surgery were distinct occupations with lineages dating to the Middle Ages. English physicians did not organize themselves as a craft guild. They did not see themselves as practicing a manual skill, as did the surgeons, or a trade, as did the apothecaries (see Berlant 1975, 132–34; Elliott 1972). With an occupational program lauding their special cognitive qualities, the Royal College of Physicians won an exclusive and unique jurisdiction from the Crown over the practice of medicine in 1511. The Royal College was generally hostile to surgeons and apothecaries, defining both as belonging to lower social strata. The Royal College attempted to subordinate each to its own general jurisdiction in a hierarchical division of labor (Berlant 1975, 132–44; see also Esland 1980, 241).

European surgeons generally held the social status of craft workers prior to the nineteenth century. In order to pursue their occupational program, British surgeons joined the barbers' guild in the 1400s. They amalgamated to form the Barber-Surgeons Guild in 1540, although barbers and surgeons held separate task jurisdictions from one another within the guild. In 1511, surgeons in Amsterdam joined the shoemakers' guild in order to serve their occupational interests (Berlant 1975, 32; Elliott 1972). Indeed, prior to the middle of the nineteenth century, the true handicraft skills demanded of the manual trades may have been superior in producing surgical results than those that surgeons actually developed. Robert T. Morris (1935, 150) tells a story of a Russian cobbler who, after stealing the license of a deceased surgeon, began a new career operating in the Kiev hospital. He completed over six hundred operations, and his mortality rate was much lower than the average for the legitimately licensed surgeons there. This cobbler rose to the rank of chief surgeon before his crime and true vocation were discovered. The key to his success, Morris argues, was in the "brutal rapidity" with which his skilled hands worked.

Prior to the nineteenth century, surgeons' own occupational skills did not win cognitive or normative legitimation from either the Church or the university (Carr-Saunders and Wilson 1933, 16, 68–69). Surgeons were constantly threatened by physicians who attempted either to subordinate them or to exclude them from medical practice altogether. In France, the Faculty of Medicine argued in the mid eighteenth century that surgeons should be excluded from physicians' training regimens because the time and unique practices required for honing surgeons' handicraft skills left them with little resources for scientific study (Russell 1966, 48).

Although the United States historically had no medical or surgical guilds, the occupational program initially adopted by the AMA lauded the omni-competent general practitioner and promoted an egalitarian ethos among physicians. As Rosemary Stevens has noted, the AMA was leery of specialization and its potential for fragmenting its jurisdiction. Consequently, the profession placed few formal restrictions on practice. Historically, physicians have been free in the United States to offer any treatments, including major surgery, they have felt competent to provide. The AMA fought against specialty licensing. Although the AMA recognized specialties in the late 1800s, the accepted model was a research association, not an association granting exclusive specialty jurisdictions (see Stevens 1971, 46–52).

Surgeons advanced their status position within the medical profession by embracing an applied "cut-and-try," craft-based orientation to new scientific discoveries. Surgeons used such discoveries in very practical ways to improve and carefully document their results (Stevens 1971, 46; see also Russell 1966, 43). The Scottish surgeon, John Hunter, pioneered the development of this form of "scientific" surgery in the eighteenth century. With the privilege of direct access to the internal organs, Hunter attempted to study the functioning of anatomy and its pathology, as well as treat it. He set about to test theories of pathology, to document empirically surgical outcomes, and to build up the knowledge base required to improve them. Hunter's scientific approach played a pivotal role in advancing surgery's status in Great Britain, in winning support from physicians for the Royal College of Surgeons, and in winning surgery's full integration into British medicine (Stevens 1986, 84; see, also, Berlant 1975, 75; Carr-Saunders and Wilson 1933, 73–75, 83; Cartwright 1967, 195; Larson 1977, 87; on the impact of this orientation on modern industry, see Braverman 1974).

This type of applied, practical orientation to scientific discoveries revolutionized surgical practice in the United States during the latter decades of the nineteenth century. After knowledge of the beneficial effects of anesthetics became widely known, and after surgeons began to use ether effectively as an anesthetic, surgical skills improved. This innovation allowed surgeons to slow down, work with deliberation, and hone their techniques (CJS 1992, 536; Morris 1935, 67). After Joseph Lister's pioneering research, following the germ theory principles developed by Louis Pasteur, uncovered the bacterial sources of infection antiseptic and aseptic techniques were developed and their use became widespread. Surgery became a viable treatment option when preventative measures against infection were employed during operations. Such practical applications of scientific developments ushered in the era of modern surgery in the United States (AnnS 1985; Shryock 1979 [1974], 176–77, 279–81). By the middle of the twentieth century, mortality and morbidity rates in every major elective category of surgery had been reduced dramatically, as surgeons worked to develop, routinize, and generalize their techniques and as they created institutional means for transmitting their skills to one another and to new generations (Surg 1983b, 122; 1990, 71). As surgeons documented their successes, surgical markets expanded.

At the time, internal medicine could not sport comparable treatment outcomes. Where surgery's successes came from direct observation in the open body cavity through trial-and-error approaches and through inductive reasoning, medicine was a cognitive discipline developing at a distance from the biophysiological processes it attempted to control. The approaches popular in the eighteenth and nineteenth centuries were deduced from theoretical conceptual systems that located pathologies in humors thought to afflict the body generally.

Take, for example, the treatment of appendicitis in the early to mid 1800s; it was a condition that was often fatal at the time. The major symptom for this condition was acute pain in the lower right side of the abdomen. Internists treated the condition with morphine, a drug that did little more than kill pain. This treatment was guided by a theory of pathology linking the condition to humors that had to run their course. The source of this condition's true pathology was localized in the anatomy, however, through autopsies indicating ruptured appendices as the cause of death. A London surgeon, Henry Hancock, treated appendicitis surgically in 1848 by removing the inflamed organ before it had the chance to rupture and kill his patient. This relatively simple operation was a tremendous success and became routinized in the latter decades of the nineteenth century (Shryock 1979 [1974], 173).

The open gallbladder procedure is often depicted in the surgical literature as the shining example of the superiority of open surgery over medical treatment. Open gallbladder surgery was first conducted by Carl Langenbuch, a German surgeon, in 1882. The procedure became standard in the United States by the 1920s (SCNA 1994d and other articles in issue). Nonsurgical treatments have developed for dissolving gallstones for patients who cannot have surgery. However, the malfunctioning organ itself forms gallstones, and the recurrence rate for stones after medical treatment has stood at about 50 percent. When surgeons incapacitate and remove the malfunctioning gallbladder the patient is cured completely and, after recovery, returns to normal functioning. Without a malfunctioning gallbladder, the recurrence rate is zero.

In the early twentieth century, in response to surgery's quantifiable treatment successes, medical internists generally ceded to surgeons control over the treatment of those conditions for which anatomical reconstruction proved superior. The occupational program that surgeons embraced to advance their interests was eventually defined as acceptable to the interests of all practicing medicine. Surgery expanded its work domain greatly in the late 1800s and the early decades of the twentieth century (Stevens 1986, 84–86; see also Morris 1935, 126; NEJM 1965). Of surgery's successes, Samuel Gross, a leading Philadelphia surgeon during the 1880s (quoted in Stevens 1986, 85) said, "Progress stares us everywhere in the face. The surgical profession was never so busy as it is at the present moment; never so fruitful in great and beneficent results, or in bold and daring exploits. . . . Operative surgery challenges the respect and admiration of the world."

Surgery's favored position in U.S. medicine is evidenced by the simple fact that rates of surgery in the United States for major categories of disease have been much higher historically than in other developed countries. Aggressive surgical treatment had become one of U.S. medicine's distinguishing characteristics by the middle of the twentieth century (ArchS 1982a).

The surgical profession established independent specialty organizations early on to pursue its occupational interests (Stevens 1971, 116–18). The American College of Surgeons (ACS) was charted in 1912. The ACS operated independently of the AMA's surgical section, as well as of the more research-oriented American Surgical Association. More so than the other organizations, the ACS attempted to regulate surgical practice. The ACS set minimum training standards for all of its members (see Hollingsworth 1986, 101–105; Stevens 1971, 87–92; Shryock 1979 [1974], 280–81). It attempted early on to halt the practice of fee-splitting between general practitioners and surgeons, a practice thought to undermine the status of surgery. It also attempted to stop "untrained" physicians from performing surgery (Stevens 1971, 124–28). In 1913, the ACS rationalized hospital practice. To attain ACS approval, a hospital was required to meet strict standards for staffing, record keeping, and facilities. The publication of the ACS listing of approved hospitals forced widespread, and much needed, reform throughout the United States (Larson 1977, 165; Shryock 1979 [1974], 280–81). Franklin Martin, the dynamic president of the ACS, became the only physician selected to serve on the Advisory Commission of the Council for National Defense during World War I. In doing so he became the national spokesperson for the medical profession (Stevens 1971, 124–28). This signaled surgery's ascendance to a dominant position in the medical profession's internal division of labor.

The profession as a whole profited from surgery's successes in treating abdominal conditions like appendicitis, stomach ulcers, and gallbladder disease. While surgeons expanded their markets as a result, nonsurgeons still provided most of the care. A normative order emerged from these developments within which medicine and surgery established and maintained a working jurisdictional balance between those patient conditions requiring medical or surgical treatment. Pathological conditions were labeled as either surgical or medical, and general practitioners directed patients to the appropriate medical or surgical specialists for diagnosis and/or treatment, accordingly. Although during this period contests for control certainly materialized over conditions that overlapped these jurisdictional boundaries, an empiricist logic and rhetoric adjudicated these contests, as each faction attempted to produce the quantifiable results needed to claim treatment superiority. Surgery competed successfully here. And surgeons were quite happy to leave those cases that could not be cured through anatomical reconstruction to others.

The initial development of the scope technology, a technology that later played a role in threatening surgical markets and in disrupting this established order, took place in the period when surgeons held a dominant position in the medical division of labor. Surgeons, by and large, accepted the endoscope as beneficial to medicine but left its development in the hands of other specialties. To understand this, we must examine more closely the general cultural frame that orients surgeons' responses to workplace innovations.

Surgeons' Definitional Frame

The distinctive time spans involved in carrying out their core tasks, for the most part, generate the distinctive cultural orientations of medical internists and surgeons (Coser 1958, 1962). Surgery involves the application of a precise anatomical manipulation that aims to "restore function and/or to cure disease" (Wechsler 1976, 26). Its success is dependent upon an in-the-moment performance. The time span from decision to action in surgery is almost instantaneous. In contrast, decision and action are more loosely coupled when medical internists perform their tasks. Internists have more time at their disposal to study their patients before they decide definitively upon a treatment course. This allows for a number of practices, such as elaborate diagnostic testing and multispecialty consultations, that are impractical for the operating room. This critical difference is acknowledged in surgical and academic commentary, such as the following:

> In other specialties you can study the patient another day or another week. You can even study the patient to death. Or to bankruptcy. When you have to balance objectives and make a decision not only whether or not to operate, but in the course of that operation if a crisis develops you have to decide instantaneously on inadequate data which way you are going to go and the patient's life quite literally hangs in the balance, that's a great responsibility. . . . The surgeon must successfully sweep aside the non-essential and decide what it is

that has to be done and go ahead and do it. (Quoted in AJS 1987c, 565; see also AnnS 1969, 650)

A number of values become lauded in the surgeons' culture in response to demands inherent in embracing a handicraft skill whose outcomes are realized through an in-the-moment performance. The internists' penchant for caution, elaborate testing, and consultation are all devalued in favor of quick thinking, decisiveness in the face of extreme stress and uncertainty, and a belief in one's own personal efficacy (see, for example, AnnS 1963a, 1967; Surg 1966, 1973b, 1974; see also Bosk 1979, 29–30; Cassell 1991; Coser 1958, 1962; Freidson 1970b, 128–30; Katz 1985, 155; Rosengren and DeVault 1963). Although clinical responsibility is highly valued in all of medicine (see Becker et al. 1961; Freidson 1970a), this value is individualized to an extreme in surgery. The surgeon takes sole responsibility in the operating room for the life-or-death outcomes delivered there. Unlike with internists, the surgeon's contribution to these outcomes is definitive; its consequences are shouldered alone. Commentaries like the following convey this attitude: "Here, at the operation, he is alone—with only the knowledge he brought to the table with him" (Surg 1974, 148); and, "For all the talk of team effort, operating is a solo activity, all the more so when speedy action is required" (ArchS 1989a, 532; see also Surg 1968b, 587).

As Howard Becker and associates (1961), Eliot Freidson (1970b), H. Jamous and B. Peloille (1970), and others (see Bosk 1979; Hoff and McCaffrey 1996) have noted, clinical practitioners define their work as involving particularistic dimensions. Surgeons embrace this view wholeheartedly. In their definitional frame, surgery's unique in-the-moment performance skills do not lend themselves to precise quantification and replication, even though their outcomes do. As with all medicine, the surgeon's subject matter—human tissue as affected by the interaction of complex physiological processes—is to some extent variable. The surgeon must recognize this and judgment must be applied on a case-by-case basis. This point is frequently noted in medical commentary (AJS 1987c, 564; see also AJS 1971b, 220; 1988d, 632; AnnS 1963a, 741).

The surgical tasks performed in the operating room are quite distinct from those valued in the internists' culture. As a handicraft, surgery demands manual skills. The operating-room performance involves uncertainty, and the types of skills valued in the handicrafts to handle such contingencies are lauded by surgeons. These include manual dexterity with both hands (AJS 1964, 671), quickness, physical stamina, and strength (AJS 1964; 1965c, 35; AnnS 1963a, 741; 1980b, 388; ArchS 1971c, 234; BJS 1986, 1; 1987b; 1991b, 1156; Surg 1969). Without good manual technique, surgical outcomes are compromised.

Acquiring these handicraft skills involves a further particularistic dimension not found in nonsurgical disciplines. Each treatment mastered must be done so in a particular way to suit each practitioner's unique physical, cognitive, and psychological characteristics. Because so much of the outcome is dependent on handicraft skills applied during a unique in-the-moment performance, surgeons tailor their procedures as an extension of their own personal particularities. The following surgical commentary sums this up:

> In surgery, as in life, all of us have and express different personalities. We, therefore, develop the various surgical procedures to fit into our own interpretation of a particular problem, its solution, our personal peculiarities and even our technical skills or limitations. Thus, many times several surgeons will attack the same problem in different ways yet end up in the same place. There is no "only way" and, in fact, few "best ways," in surgery. (AJS 1965b, 61)

Because of surgery's particularistic foundation, surgical skills develop only through experience in apprenticeship training (AJS 1988d, 632; AnnS 1967, 307; BJS 1986; Surg 1974; see also Bosk 1979, 13). Surgical residency programs have many characteristics in common with the apprenticeships found in industrial crafts. Rather than relying on standardized texts, for example, surgical educators encourage residents to log their personal operating experiences in diaries for future reference whenever they encounter similar circumstances. This enables surgeons-in-training to particularize their working references so that they can be used most effectively (AJS 1987b, 424; Surg 1989, 587). This type of black-book logging is quite common in industrial crafts, such as in mechanical repair, metal machining, and the tool-and-die trade (see Noble 1984; Shaiken 1984).

Thus, the demands inherent in an in-the-moment performance, whose consequences can be measured in terms of a life-and-death calculus and attributed to a single responsible agent, gives rise to a distinctive occupational culture. This culture values individualism, decisiveness, quick thinking, a strong ego, and manual dexterity. It embraces particularism in the extreme, and transmits its values through classic hands-on apprenticeship training.

Surgeons' Response to Workplace Developments

Surgeons respond to the difficult workplace demands they confront day in and day out by transforming their operating theater into extensions of their particularistic egos—extensions they control unilaterally (ArchS 1971a, 104; CJS 1994b, 8). The obsessiveness with which surgeons assert such control is noted in both medical and surgical commentary. It reflects the precariousness inherent in the act of opening up another human being's body in order to do good, as well as the enormous responsibility felt by the surgeon who engages in this act day in and day out. The following commentary captures it:

> Who better than the surgeon is aware of the awesome responsibility which is his when a trusting patient places his life in his hands, when a split-second decision in the operating room, a move of the hand, may make the difference between life and death, between robust health and lifelong disability? It is not surprising that to many surgeons their calling becomes almost a religion with the operating suite the temple for their devotions. (AJS 1977a, 3)

Any threat to the practices, routines, and rituals a surgeon establishes to control his or her operating room performance is defined in the surgeons' culture as sacrilege. "Don't mess around in my temple," is the crudely put defining motif of surgeons' orientation to workplace change. And surgeons have resisted changes that have stood to disrupt their operating-room control. This is the part of the work domain that surgeons define as their core domain. It is here where they apply their core skills and demonstrate their occupational virtue to others. However, it must be remembered that operating-room tasks are only a fraction of the total bundle of tasks surgeons' perform. In addition to what they do in the operating room, surgeons engage in numerous presurgical and postsurgical activities. In these areas, surgeons have routinely embraced and encouraged innovations, as such innovations typically are nonthreatening to their core operating-room skills.

Surgery and Anesthesiology

Surgeons' initial responses to the development of anesthesiology as a medical specialty illustrates the surgeons' workplace orientation quite well. Surgeons have generally delegated control over both the introduction of anesthetics and the monitoring of the patient under their influence to nonsurgical personnel. Such delegation is functional to surgeons' control over their core tasks, because it frees them to concentrate their attention and effort on the operation at hand. This delegation traditionally had no effect on the surgeons' unilateral authority in the operation room, because nurses administered anesthetics and accepted a subordinate role there.

However, as the knowledge base involved in administering anesthetics gained complexity, anesthesiology was organized and formally recognized by the Advisory Board for Medical Specialties, first as an affiliate of the American Board of Surgery in 1938, then as an independent specialty in 1941 (Stevens 1971, 238–42). Thereafter, anesthesiologists generally attempted to take control over their own core tasks, tasks that they happened to perform in the operating room alongside the surgeons. While the surgeon remained in sole control over actual operating tasks, anesthesiologists claimed joint responsibility for drugs used to control patients' blood and fluid levels, for the particular anesthetic administered, for the supervision of the nurse, and for administrative functions (Surg 1981a, 1981b). And anesthesiologists, as members of a hungry and relatively new specialty, did not readily submit to the surgeons' authority claims over those functions for which they themselves held expertise.

Some surgeons chafed at this development, defining it as an untoward encroachment on their sacred temple. Operating-room conflicts between the specialties were frequent; they found expression in surgical commentary (Surg 1981a, 1981b). For example, a general surgeon stated in commentary:

> To the surgeon, this unprecedented challenge to his traditional position has been truly intolerable; the responsibility remains his, but the authority has vanished. He can control all other personnel but must negotiate with the anesthesiologist. To surgical nurses and technicians, the situation has been confusing and, at times, demoralizing. . . . Dual command, impractical on a battleship, is equally so in the operating room. (SGO 1971, 887)

Echoing commonly shared sentiments, this surgeon championed the replacement of the anesthesiologist with the nurse anesthetician. This would restore the traditional authority relationship in the operating room, inasmuch as the nurse was trained to submit to surgeons' unilateral authority. In the spirit of a call to arms he also stated:

> It becomes increasingly clear that, sooner or later, a stand will have to be made; the present anarchic state is unacceptable. The longer it is delayed, the more difficult it will be to dislodge an opponent more deeply entrenched. It, therefore, now seems necessary that surgeons . . . take whatever steps are needed to return to their traditional and rightful place as the sole authority in the operating room. (SGO 1971, 888)

This militant response is best interpreted as a reaction to the threat of dual authority to surgeons' tightly coupled operating room routines. Such a response, however, was not universal. Other personnel changes, in fact, did not appear from my review of the surgical commentary to generate such reaction. In the 1970s, for example, some hospitals began training and using nursing personnel—rather than M.D.s—as surgical assistants. Surgical commentary regarding this trend was generally favorable (AJS 1970, 1976c; AnnS 1981a; ArchS 1976; Surg 1978c). Unlike the development of anesthesiologists, specialized surgical assistants did not threaten surgeons' unilateral operating-room authority.

Surgery and the Early Scopes

Although general surgeons did embrace the videoscope in the early 1990s, they were rather indifferent to the endoscope's prevideo developments. Diagnostic laparoscopy, a technique employed by some gastroenterologists since the 1960s (AJG 1962; Gas 1976c; see, also, AJS 1975b; SCNA 1992) and virtually all surgical gynecologists since the early 1970s (AJOG 1970; COG 1976; JRM 1976), was not embraced by general surgeons on a notable scale until the 1990s. Of course, accurate diagnosis is important to surgery, and a pattern evolved from the days of surgery's "Golden Age" that enabled surgeons to incorporate the results of a host of diagnostic tests into their decision-making routines. For nonemergency cases, surgeons typically delegated diagnostic testing to nonsurgical specialties, such as internal medicine, gastroenterology, and radiology. Surgeons let others perform this function and then incorporated their recommendations into their presurgical assessments.

However, in emergency cases surgeons appropriated this function. They initiated exploratory surgery, opening the belly and examining the inner abdomen with direct vision and feel. Here, surgeons accepted a nonincidence rate of 20 percent or higher so as not to miss an urgent, perhaps life threatening, surgical condition (AmS 1986; see also Nolen 1970, 58). Exploratory laparotomies no doubt saved many patients. However, those patients who were not afflicted with conditions requiring surgery suffered mightily from the iatrogenic consequences of unnecessary open surgery.

When they finally embraced the videoscope in the 1990s, surgeons began to realize that the costs that patients paid for their exploratory surgeries in the past were largely unnecessary (AJS 1991b, 1991c; see also SGO 1977). Laparoscopy could have been used effectively long before as an alternative. This method provided an excellent view of the inner abdomen without the large incision required for open access. If surgery was not indicated by the diagnostic laparoscopy, the condition could be treated medically and the patient could often leave the hospital in a day or two and quickly return to work. Rather than the massive surgical wound, the patient carried from the laparoscopic procedure only a Band-Aid-sized puncture at the navel. Gynecologists, to their patients' benefit, embraced this less-invasive scope technique on a massive scale during the 1970s. Abdominal surgeons flatly refused.

A handful of pioneering general surgeons, however, did develop intraoperative uses for endoscopes long before the advent of video laparoscopy. For example, open gallbladder surgery, although enormously successful, had one significant blemish on its historical record—stones left in the biliary ducts. The reported incidence of this ranged from less than 5 to as high as 20 percent after open surgeries for gallbladder removal (AJS 1980b; AmS 1981; 1989b, 271). The consequences of retained gallstones were often severe. Patients underwent a second operation. The operative mortality rate for this was reported to be from 4 to 10 percent, much higher than for the initial gallbladder operation (AnnS 1986c, 260). Surgical commentary suggests that such cases were embarrassments to surgeons (AmS 1989b, 271).

To their credit, most surgeons did employ cholangiography during their gallbladder operations to examine the biliary ducts for stones. Cholangiography involved the insertion of radioactive fluid into the ductal system and the making of films to indicate whether stones were present. This procedure was accomplished in a few minutes. It reduced the rate of retained stones to 5 percent or less (AJS 1974a; BJS 1987a). However, there were flaws with this procedure, as made clear in the following commentary:

> Despite its value in biliary tract surgery, operative cholangiography has many limitations. Very often it fails to demonstrate the presence of stones in the bile ducts due to poor quality of films and the super-imposition of adjacent organs. Air bubbles, blood clots, artifacts and fibrinous materials may be confused with stones in interpreting the cholangiogram, leading to unnecessary and time-consuming exploration of the bile ducts. (AJS 1980b, 651; see also ARCSE 1989; BJS 1987a)

In removing stones indicated by this method, surgeons searched blindly in the biliary ducts with graspers, spoons, and probes. This technique also left much to be desired (ArchS 1982b, 606; see also AmS 1989b, 267).

Not satisfied with this state of affairs, a handful of enterprising surgeons developed an intraoperative technique for biliary tract exploration using a side-viewing endoscope—the choledochoscope. This technique was developed long before the advent of video laparoscopic surgery. With the abdominal cavity open, these scopes could be inserted into the tubular biliary ducts (see, for example, AmS 1984; AnnS 1980a; BJS 1991a). Choledochoscopy promised to reduce the incidence of retained stones, as well as the risks involved in biliary surgery, because stones could be viewed directly and removed under direct vision through an operative channel in the scope. The technique, while adding operative time, was performed during gallbladder removal. It did not threaten to displace a conventional surgery nor did it, as an adjunct to gallbladder removal, threaten conventional skills. Proponents claimed the technique could reduce the rate of retained stones to 1 to 2 percent (see AJS 1976c, 1979c, 1980a, 1980b, 1984; AmS 1963, 1989b; AnnS 1981b).

Although promising, this technique was not embraced by most practitioners in general surgery. Biliary endoscopists hoped that, through constantly improving the technique, the surgical community would eventually come around. Monroe McIver, using the urologists' right-angled cystoscope, is credited with developing the first modern choledochoscope in 1941. This scope was replaced in 1953 by a rigid instrument developed by H. Wildegands from Germany (see AJS 1977c, 1990b). The Wildegands scope spread throughout Europe. It was adopted by Clarence Schein and Elliott Hurwitt in New York and by J. Manny Shore and Harvey Lippman in Los Angeles (AJS 1975a; AmS 1963; AnnS 1970; Surg 1962). However, these early instruments proved awkward to use and visualization was poor (AmS 1981, 121, 123).

Harold Hopkins revolutionized endoscopy by developing an innovative system for optical transmission that built on developments in fiber-optic technology, since referred to as the Hopkins rod-lens system. In this system flexible glass rods serve as the primary medium transmitting light through the instrument. This innovation increased light transmission and provided a superior view. It also allowed a significant reduction in the scope's diameter, thereby increasing its flexibility and enlarging its viewing angle (AmS 1972). The Hopkins rod-lens system was introduced for choledochoscopy in the United States in 1969 (AmS 1981, 123; see also AJS 1971a; 1980b, 648).

Biliary endoscopists assumed that, with the spread of this improved instrument, general surgeons would fully embrace choledochoscopy. Research evidence suggested, however, that this never happened. The published results of a 1985 study were quite discouraging. In a survey of 184 large hospitals in California, 87 percent had the instrument available in the operating room, but only 8 percent of the surgeons reported using it regularly during gallbladder operations (AJS 1985, 703–704). On surgeons' refusal to embrace this technique, endoscopic proponents stated on a frustrated note:

> Surgeons have abrogated their responsibilities of becoming proficient in endoscopy. . . . It is well recognized that surgeons generally have psychological barriers against trying new techniques or devices. By now, it is already some 14 years since biliary endoscopy in its presently developed state of excellence has been available. (AJS 1985, 703; see also AJS 1987a, 576)

However, there was more to this resistance than a psychological barrier. Initially proponents of biliary endoscopy naively underestimated the method's skill demands, assuming that the surgeon had little more to do than to insert the scope, look at the findings, and go to work (AnnS 1970, 277). The radical nature of choledochoscopy's skill demands were not appreciated, nor readily admitted by the technique's proponents, until much later.

Three of choledochoscopy's skill demands are worth mentioning. First, the use of the choledochoscope requires a shift from the direct binocular view afforded by a well-lit operating theater to the darker, nondirect image coming through the scope's eyepiece. This shift caused disorientation and made adaptation difficult (SCNA 1989b, 1277; see also ARCSE 1991, 103).

Second, the visual-spatial coordination demanded of this technique was somewhat similar to that of the video laparoscopic technique described in chapter 1. Picking up the hand-eye coordination required to maneuver the scope and the instruments threaded through it from a remote location involved a learning curve that, for many, was difficult (see ARCSE 1991, 100–103). As noted in surgical commentary, most surgeons were not endoscopists. In the typical practice surgeons did not see the number of cases required to hone the necessary skills (SCNA 1989b, 1276).

Third, with the development of extraction techniques, choledochoscopy became a two-person job, requiring close effort coordination. With choledochoscopy, the operating surgeon used two hands: one to keep the duodenum stretched while the other introduced the scope. The assistant advanced the instrument used to extract the stone through the scope. Then, the surgeon and assistant coordinated their actions closely to secure the stone and extract it (AmS 1989b, 268). The primary and assistant had to work together fluidly during choledochoscopy so that the stone could be removed without causing unnecessary inflammation of the duct. Recognizing that this difficult coordination demand was a factor inhibiting the technique's acceptance, proponents championed the use of videoscopes and television monitors in the later 1980s, believing that these would facilitate more effective teamwork (AmS 1989b, 267–72; SGO 1985).

Understanding the occupational culture of open surgery can help make sense out of surgeons' resistance to embracing techniques like choledochoscopy. The skill demands required of this technique were difficult. The technique required that surgeons shift from their favored working modality to an alien one—one that required the development of visual and manual skills very different than those mastered for open work. The group-coordination demand, moreover, was alien to surgeons' ethos of individual responsibility and control.

Innovations such as these were not welcomed. Surgeons preferred the time-honored methods they knew and thought they could control in the operating room. Anything that could disrupt that control might jeopardize the outcomes for which they were held responsible. This reluctance is not irrational. In the case of choledochoscopy, the surgeon had to assess personally whether the benefits of reducing the percentage of cases with biliary tract stones after gallbladder removal was worth the risk involved in potentially losing control over the operating theater with a new and unfamiliar technology. For most, it apparently was not.

In fact, the stereotype of a rearguard conservative quick to resist any technical change no matter what its potential benefit, is unwarranted. Surgeons have been resistant only to those technological innovations disruptive to their hands-on operating room control. They have encouraged other developments, such as the development of X-rays (AJS 1993d), fluoroscopic radiographic techniques, and even presurgical diagnostic endoscopy. Surgeons have incorporated the results produced by these technologies into their pre-operative and postoperative routines in order to improve surgical outcomes. Historically, surgeons have delegated the performance of these diagnostic techniques to others. Although surgeons recognized their usefulness, they saw them as lacking the virtue and glory inherent in true surgical work.

The distinctive cultural frame embraced by abdominal surgeons helped shape the early development of the scope technology. General surgeons were not shut off from the technology by their internist competitors; indeed, some specialties with surgical orientations, such as urology and otolaryngology, had developed a long history of using diagnostic and some surgical applications of rigid, prevideo endoscopes. Rather, with their interests riveted to their performances in the operating room, general surgeons simply chose not to play a role in the endoscope's gastrointestinal and interabdominal developments (SCNA 1992, 661–2; see also SCNA 1989a, 1129), leaving the technology to their medical counterparts, fully expecting to appropriate whatever beneficial results they accomplished with it for their own purposes in the operating room (SGO 1973). After all, this was the time-honored pattern that had won acceptance in medicine. And, it was almost inconceivable in the early years that these scopes could be used to mount a serious challenge to general surgeons' time-honored markets.

Notes

1. According to Shryock (1979 [1974], 53–54), medical faculties have viewed surgery as a mere craft since the Middle Ages.

2. For the importance of measurement and quantification in advancing medicine, see Shryock (1979 [1974]).

5

Gastroenterologists Embrace the Scope

In the mid-1950s, anyone who approached general surgeons and dared to suggest that their internist counterparts—the gastroenterologists—would threaten their market turf in the upcoming decades probably would have been laughed out of the hospital. Historically, the development of gastroenterology lagged behind that of gastrointestinal surgery. Before 1960, gastroenterologists primarily provided consultations to general practitioners regarding their patients' digestive problems and screened candidates for surgical treatment. Of gastroenterological practice then, a commentator stated, "If a digestive complaint didn't get better on its own (which it usually did), or if a pill or medical counsel couldn't relieve the symptoms, you called a surgeon, a radiotherapist, or a clergyman (Gas 1986a, 217)."

Until the advent of fiber-optic endoscopy, gastroenterology suffered from an image problem. Early gastroenterologists could not sport the documented successes of their surgical counterparts. For many years gastroenterology's knowledge base was defined as too underdeveloped to merit specialty status. Although serious gastrointestinal disorders took a considerable toll on patients' well being, such disorders often lacked the urgency and marketability of those treated by other subspecialties of internal medicine such as cardiology or oncology. Until the advent of fiber-optic endoscopy gastroenterology failed to attract much interest from medical students (Gas 1970; JAMA 1970b). One commentator defined gastroenterology's image problem as being similar to that encountered in the promotion of prunes (see Gas 1970, 338).

The first specialty association formed in the United States for the study of digestive problems was the American Gastroenterological Association (AGA), founded in 1897. Following the model sanctioned by the American Medical Association (AMA), the AGA functioned as a theoretically oriented research society. It recognized the undeveloped state of medicine's knowledge base regarding digestive disorders and devoted its efforts to learning more about its subject matter (AJG 1989; Gas 1981b, 1987). However, progress was slow. Knowledge of digestive diseases was rudimentary, and internists lacked direct access to the organ systems (Shryock 1979 [1974], 41). At a time when abdominal surgeons were documenting substantial progress, gastroenterologists could do little better than apply a general label to patients' maladies—that is, "dyspepsia"—and dispense general-purpose medicines for a variety of conditions, little understood (Gas 1993c). The AMA did not recognize gastroenterology as a subspecialty of internal medicine until 1940. The AGA did not establish its medical journal, *Gastroenterology*, until 1942. The AGA did not define itself as gastroenterologists' national spokesperson until 1967 (Gas 1981b; Stevens 1971, 214–16, 234–35).

Other associations developed to challenge the AGA's anemic leadership. In 1932 a group seeking to serve the needs of clinical practitioners specializing in gastrointestinal disorders organized the Society for the Advancement of Gastroenterology. In 1934 the Society established the first national gastroenterological journal. In 1954 the Society became the American College of Gastroenterology and its journal was renamed the *American Journal of Gastroenterology* (AJG 1983a, 1992; JAMA 1988). Another organization, devoted to advancing the work of émigré endoscopist, Rudolf Schindler, was founded in 1941 as the American Gastroscopic Club. This association was the first to champion gastrointestinal endoscopy. It later was renamed the American Society for Gastrointestinal Endoscopy (ASGE) (Gas 1981b).

Although gastrointestinal gastroscopy, an endoscopic technique used for exploring directly the upper gastrointestinal tract, can trace its origins to the late nineteenth century (BMB 1986c; Gas 1979f), Schindler pioneered the technique's modern development. Schindler began his experiments with the endoscope in Germany during the 1920s and continued them at the University of Chicago during the

1930s and 1940s (AJG 1989; Gas 1993b). Some of the early American endoscopists understudied with Schindler and used the ASGE to share their results (AJG 1979, 224; Gas 1993b). However, it took them many years to win recognition.

Prior to fiber optics, surgeons who specialized in anatomy that was difficult to access—throat surgeons, colon and rectal surgeons, and urologists—were as likely to use the rigid endoscopes as were gastroenterologists. These scopes were difficult to use deep inside the gastrointestinal tract, as evidenced in the following gastroenterologist's recollection:

> We did one or two gastroscopies each week at the hospital in which I trained [1940s]. Informed consent was primitive and consisted of telling the patient that a "flexible" tube with a light at its end would be passed down into his stomach. We did not tell him that of the three foot scope, the flexible portion measured only about 8 inches; the rest was a rigid stainless steel rod. For we feared that if the patient knew, he would refuse our attempts to help. And so, medicated with sodium phenobarbital . . . the patient was ferried to the endoscopy room where the instrument was kept hidden lest its appearance frighten him away. (AJG 1983b, 60)

Although gastroenterology needed a significant development to lay claim to status within the medical profession, this peculiar instrument left much to be desired. Most gastroenterologists did not readily embrace the early scopes. The endoscopic pioneers in gastroenterology labored in relative obscurity.

However, this situation changed dramatically after developments in fiber optics were incorporated into the design of the endoscope in the 1950s (AJG 1983b). Passing light transmission through optical glass enabled instrument manufacturers to narrow significantly the scope's diameter, to create flexible and easier to use instruments, and to improve the image transmitted. These improved instruments eventually allowed endoscopists to access all regions of the gastrointestinal tract. Gastroenterologists quickly embraced these improved instruments as their own. From 1962 on, papers pertaining to endoscopy began to dominate presentations at gastroenterologists' professional meetings. From 1976 on, these papers increasingly turned to discussions of operative endoscopy, especially laser therapy (AJG 1986b).

Fiber-optic endoscopy revitalized and reshaped gastroenterology. The discipline began to attract unprecedented interest from new M.D.s eager to make their mark on medicine. The attractiveness of this new technology was frequently noted in gastroenterological commentary (Gas 1992b, 1715; see also Gas 1976b, 540; AJG 1983b, 60).

Embracing Endoscopy within the Internists' Definitional Frame

Unlike the endoscopic specialties that developed in surgery—urology, gynecology, and otolaryngology—gastroenterology never established full independence. It holds status as a subspecialty within the general specialty of internal medicine. As such, gastroenterologists must first become certified in internal medicine before they train exclusively in their chosen field (Gas 1967a, 1977, 1992b). The American Board of Internal Medicine (ABIM) emphasizes in its guidelines for subspecialist training the importance of developing a wide knowledge base, understanding the subspecialty's relationship to the whole of internal medicine, and maintaining a broad clinical practice (ArchS 1987; Gas 1979d). Gastroenterologists are thoroughly socialized into internal medicine's worldview and values during their residency training. In addition to consultations with other physicians, the AGA encourages gastroenterologists to provide broad primary care (Gas 1980a, 955). And gastroenterologists apparently do so. The president of the ABIM, in addressing the AGA convention in 1978, reported that gastroenterologists were providing primary care to patients and that gastroenterologists were treating approximately 40 percent of their patients for chronic, multiple problems. Gastroenterologists also referred out more of their patients for treatment to specialists (Gas 1978b). Gastroenterologists' multifaceted role in medicine as both specialists and general internists is often mentioned in commentary (Gas 1981a, 861; 1993a, 1563; see also AJG 1986b, 213; 1993e, 330; Gas 1976b, 539).

As noted previously, internists' culture is markedly different than that of surgeons. The "science" of surgery was built inductively from the ground up. It developed from clinical surgeons' hands-on successes in the abdominal cavity and from the careful documentation and replication of these successes. Lacking direct access to functioning organ systems and to the biophysiological processes affecting them, internists worked first to build up their theoretical knowledge. They then developed strategies for using this abstract knowledge base to treat cases more effectively. Practice largely followed theory.

Gastroenterologists are internists. As such, they define accurately diagnosing patients' conditions, prior to treatment, as their core clinical task. The skills they value are cognitive in nature, primarily deductive. Internists correlate patients' particular complaints and conditions with their theoretical understanding of biophysiological processes. As Paul Atkinson reports, Conan Doyle modeled the skills of his famous fictional detective, Sherlock Holmes, on the inferential practices typical of medical internists (Atkinson 1981, 115–16; see also Atkinson 1971, 31; Wechsler 1976, 116–17). Lauding diagnostic prowess, subspecialists in internal medicine typically delegate the prescription and monitoring of treatment regimens to others.

Accepting the internists' definition of medicine's core skill, as well as the normatively regulated division of labor that had long been established between medicine and surgery, gastroenterologists embraced the first fiber-optic scopes as diagnostic tools. With these tools, gastroenterologists for the first time could examine directly the functioning organs they studied, diagnosed, and sometimes treated. This allowed them to sharpen and expand their theoretical understanding. This promised better diagnosis and far greater accuracy in locating the source of difficulties in the gastrointestinal tract. Better diagnosis, it was thought, could better screen surgical from medical patients, help treatment decisions, and aid surgeons in their work. Who could oppose the advancement of such a promising tool? Early efforts to develop gastroenterological endoscopy were quite acceptable to the interests of the established guard in gastroenterology, internal medicine, and surgery. As an aid to presurgical diagnosis, scopes were not threatening to the established demarcation of medical and surgical turf.

New Skill Demands

To legitimate their efforts to incorporate endoscopic practices into their routines, gastrointestinal endoscopists stressed that the cognitive and interpretive foundation of successful endoscopy built upon the theoretical knowledge base established in traditional gastro-enterology (AJG 1984a). However, while drawing from the same theoretical foundation, and while employing similar cognitive and interpretive skills in diagnosing cases, the introduction of endoscopy did involve significant changes in gastroenterologists' work orientation and practice. These changes, in fact, shifted gastroenterologists' action orientation somewhat closer to that of surgeons.

First, doing endoscopy requires a thorough understanding of the case-by-case nuances of anatomy. This type of fine-grained experiential knowledge base was not used by traditional gastroenterologists who interpreted conditions indirectly from information elicited through physician-patient interaction and through physical exams. Second, the understanding of anatomy required for successful endoscopy is built up through direct experience looking directly at tissue in all of its empirical manifestations. As in surgery, this type of understanding is appropriated by each individual endoscopist in a particularistic way (AJG 1993a; for a critique of this, see AJG 1993b). Third, as in surgery, successful endoscopy involves manual skills that are put into effect during an in-the-moment performance. The most important and fundamental of these manual skills is physically passing the scope from its access port to the desired location inside the gastrointestinal tract (SCNA 1982a, 870). Endoscopy is invasive. Organ ruptures and perforations, although rare, are documented risks (see, for example, AJG 1978a, 318; AJS 1977b; JAMA 1977c). Such risks are minimized through the development of handicraft skill (see, for example, Gas 1976a).

These performance skills hold peculiarities distinct from those involved in open surgery, nonetheless. Although the scope directly accesses the tissue of interest, endoscopists work from a remote location at the orifice that serves as the instrument's port—in the case of gastroenterological work, the patient's mouth or anus. Endoscopists manipulate a variety of mechanisms at the base of the endoscope from these remote locations to guide the light source or camera and the various types of tools threaded through the scope's channels. There is no tactile sensation or direct control of tissue as in surgery. Most importantly, the gastrointestinal endoscopist accesses tissue from within the organ system, while the surgeon accesses tissue from the outside through the abdominal wall. Adjusting to the work demands of this remote environment takes time, effort, and repeated experience (SCNA 1982a, 869).

Early Diagnostic Successes

The physicians entering gastroenterological fellowship programs in the late 1960s and early 1970s readily embraced the new endoscopes. They used these instruments in the way they were intended—to improve the diagnosis of medical and surgical conditions in the gastrointestinal tract. By the middle 1970s considerable successes had been reported. First, gastroscopes were used to locate and diagnose bleeding sources. Studies reported documented success rates as high as 96 percent (AJS 1979a; ArchS 1978b), compared to a success rate with earlier radiographic techniques of from 50 to 60 percent (Gas 1976b, 540). Second, channels were soon built into the scopes to pass instruments for biopsy and for brush cytology, and this aided gastroenterologists in distinguishing between benign and malignant gastrointestinal tumors prior to surgery (JAMA 1970a). Third, gastroenterologists used their endoscopes during emergency bleeding to pinpoint the specific vessel responsible. If such a vessel could be visualized, surgery was recommended immediately, and the endoscopic findings aided the surgeon's efforts in quickly locating and repairing the bleeding source. If a visible vessel was not found, the condition was treated medically (NEJM 1979b).

Successes were also reported in the lower gastrointestinal tract. The colonoscope was used first as an adjunct to radiographic studies to localize bleeding sources in the colon (AJS 1979b, 627; see also JAMA 1971). Shortly thereafter, it was used to locate lesions and polyps, to define whether such tissues were benign or malignant, and in some cases to allow patients to avoid costly exploratory surgeries (BMB 1986b, 265; JAMA 1971). Endoscopic methods, coupled with radiological techniques, were also pioneered that allowed for the presurgical visualization of the pancreatic and biliary ducts. These findings provided surgeons with precise preoperative data (AnnS 1973).

These successes bolstered gastroenterology's status. The scope proved to be a great diagnostic aid. As a gastroenterological commentary proclaimed in 1975, "Gastrointestinal endoscopy is recognized as the single most important advance in the diagnosis of diseases of the gastrointestinal tract that has been introduced in the last 15 years (Gas 1975, 1308)."

Pockets of Resistance and Endoscopists' Responses

Despite these successes, it was not long before endoscopy's place in gastroenterological practice was challenged. The first challenge came from within the gastroenterological ranks themselves and was easily dealt with. Endoscopists argued that their instruments delivered the goods long valued in the internists' culture—accurate diagnoses. However, the second challenge questioned the ultimate value of internists' self-defined core skill—delivering accurate diagnoses—to patient care. Rather than slow endoscopy's development, however, this challenge spurred endoscopists to reject the traditional turf demarcation line between gastrointestinal medicine and surgery and to embrace operative endoscopic applications. With this move, gastroenterologists began to invade general surgeons' time-honored markets.

Internal Resistance

Historically, there is no counterpart in the internists' bundle of tasks to surgeons' craft-based, in-the-moment performance skills. Accurately assessing the case, deducing its biophysiological causes, and determining the most effective treatment are not approached within the internists' culture as time-bound performances. Getting it right, it is thought, requires a flexible time span for thinking, consultation, and even some trial-and-error experimentation. However, fiber-optic endoscopy introduced a tool to the internists' diagnostic arsenal that demanded in-the-moment performance skills. While the generation flocking to gastroenterological fellowship programs in the 1960s and 1970s readily embraced endoscopy, some among the older generation questioned both the necessity of having gastroenterologists performing this difficult technique, as well as its impact on the specialty's development.

In fact, some within the older generation, being deeply committed to the internists' occupational culture, grew increasingly hostile to the endoscope. The scope, from their point of view, was undermining the cognitive foundation of the specialty, turning gastroenterologists into little more than technicians. This voice was rather strong. One commentator, for example, lamented what he saw as the rapid deterioration of the time-honored skills of history taking, interviewing patients, and deduction (Gut 1990, 125–26). Another saw the preoccupation with technical aspects of endoscopy as undermining young gastroenterologists' theoretical depth (NEJM 1977c). Summing up the older generation's frustration, Dr. Fred Kern (Gas 1979a, 1490; see also NEJM 1977b) stated in his presidential address to the American Gastroenterological Association:

> [Gastroenterological fellows] devote a major portion of their time to performing procedures, primarily endoscopy, instead of to activities that would produce scholarly and thoughtful consultants: talking to their patients, learning (by doing) clinical physiology, reading in the library and thinking. . . . I bitterly resent [endoscopy's] effects on the training of generations of gastroenterologists and on the values of many young gastroenterologists.

Some critics, like Dr. Kern, had a remedy. This involved establishing a division of labor between "true" gastroenterologists, who would function in a traditional role as theoretical consultants on digestive diseases, and technicians, who would perform the more routinized endoscopic tasks. As championed by Dr. Kern (Gas 1979a, 1979e), the latter could be non-M.D.s, especially for the easier procedures. Perhaps even radiologists, whose techniques were threatened by endoscopy, could be candidates for the technician's role.

Endoscopists were quick to answer this criticism in commentary. First, endoscopists argued that their technique actually delivered the goods valued most in the internist's culture—accurate diagnoses. They pointed to endoscopy's documented successes in improving diagnostic accuracy as the technology's ultimate justification. As stated in one gastroenterological commentary, "The emphasis in clinical training today on endoscopy is so because accurate diagnosis before treatment, and nonsurgical treatment wherever possible is what other physicians demand of gastroenterologists and what we demand of ourselves (Gas 1979b, 1163; see also AJG 1979; JAMA 1980a)." Such commentators also pointed to the growing job market for endoscopists as proof, in itself, of their technique's value (NEJM 1977c).

Second, gastroenterological endoscopists challenged the assumption that adding a performance-based skill to their diagnostic armamentarium would somehow cheapen their status as theoretically oriented internists. They argued that, because endoscopy demanded cognitive and interpretive skills both during the procedure and afterward in assessing the significance of the findings, it was best to have gastroenterologists doing it. They argued that other highly regarded specialties used manual tools and techniques without hurting their theoretical status (NEJM 1977a, 1406; see also Gas 1979b, 1979c).

Finally, an appeal was made to the reality of intraoccupational competition. One commentator, for example, fingered the criticisms of endoscopy as the feeble cries of practitioners out of touch and out of date, facing losses befitting those who refuse to embrace the march of technological progress (Gas 1979b). Another expressed fear that, if gastroenterologists delegated the scope, severe market consequences would result (Gas 1979a, 1492).

Of course, the critiques from within the subspecialty did not prevail. Gastroenterology has embraced a strong technical-procedural orientation since the 1970s. Its contemporary practice demands proficiency in a variety of endoscopic techniques. The American Society for Gastrointestinal Endoscopy established minimum guidelines for demonstrating competency in gastroenterological endoscopy. These guidelines stipulated the performance of one hundred endoscopies of the upper gastrointestinal tract, fifty colonoscopies, twenty-five polypectomies, twenty-five endoscopic retrograde cholangiopancreatographies (ERCPs), and twenty-five laparoscopies (AJG 1979, 226). Although these guidelines drew criticism from a number of camps— for example, from residency directors who could not provide the number of cases to meet them, from practitioners who saw only a limited application for ERCP and laparoscopy in their practices, and from academic gastroenterologists who believed that skill and cognitive mastery should take precedence over simple procedural counts—they were picked up by hospitals seeking reasonable criteria for granting privileges (AJG 1987c).

In 1977, the ABIM published guidelines for training gastroenterologists that emphasized the growing importance of procedural skills to this subspecialty (AJG 1981, 1987c; see also Gas 1977, 1978b; for guideline criticism see AJG 1987a; Gas 1980b). In 1983 the Liaison Committee on Graduate Medical Education authorized the Residency Review Committee in Internal Medicine to review its sub-specialty programs for their compliance with published training guidelines. The guideline that was accepted recognized the importance of endoscopy to gastroenterological training. A specific appendix for endoscopic training was included in the statement. The statement placed the responsibility for assessing residents' endoscopic skills in the hands of residency program directors. The Training and Education Committee of the AGA adopted a position statement that similarly emphasized the importance of procedural skills to the practice of clinical endoscopy (Gas 1987).

Indeed, by the 1980s gastroenterologists were spending a considerable amount of their time performing endoscopic procedures. A membership survey sponsored by the AGA found that academic faculty reported spending one-third of their time on patient care for gastrointestinal problems, and an additional 15 percent of their time performing endoscopic procedures. Nonfaculty members reported spending 56 percent of their time on patient care, and an additional 22 percent of their time performing endoscopic procedures (Gas 1986b; see also AJG 1989, 230). Endoscopy had also become a major component of gastroenterological consultations. A 1976 study of consultations performed by gastroenterologists practicing in the Denver area found that 60 percent of patients were referred for procedures, and that 60 to 65 percent of these procedures were endoscopies (Gas 1976b). Endoscopic procedures had become even more important to gastroenterologists' revenue stream. A 1991 study reported that, while making up only 17.6 percent of the services billed by gastroenterologists, endoscopies generated 66.6 percent of the total charges billed (AJG 1991). By the 1980s, endoscopy had won a very secure place in gastroenterology.

Challenge to Diagnostic Acumen as the Core Medical Virtue

Critics mounted a more formidable challenge to gastroenterological endoscopy at the end of the 1970s. This challenge did not revoke the claims that endoscopists made regarding their diagnostic successes—it accepted these claims as completely valid. Rather, the critics of endoscopy questioned the ultimate value of more accurate diagnosis to improving patient outcomes, a questioning that directly challenged the internists' core skill.

Such criticism appeared warranted. Studies published in the late

1970s and early 1980s showed that scoped patients suffering from upper gastrointestinal bleeding, even when diagnosed more accurately, showed no appreciable difference from those patients who were not scoped in terms of mortality rates, recurrence rates, the amount of transfusions required, or the frequency of surgery (NEJM 1981c; see also AJS 1980c; JAMA 1985; NEJM 1981b, 1982c). Some commentators argued that the risks associated with endoscopy—small but statistically significant—were not worth the procedure's potential benefits without documented improvements in bottom-line treatment results (NEJM 1981c, 925–29; see also NEJM 1982b). Similar arguments were made against colonoscopy as a presurgical technique for diagnosing cancer in patients with long-term colitis (JAMA 1976a, 1977b). Both American and British radiologists used such arguments to champion the less accurate but cheaper and less invasive radiological techniques threatened by the endoscope (for the British response, see, for example, Lancet 1985a, 1985b; for the American response, see Gas 1976d).

Some of the immediate gastroenterological commentary in response to these claims was quite defensive (see AJG 1978c, 534). However, if gastroenterologists were to continue to embrace the scope, they would have to justify its efficacy in terms of its ultimate benefit to patient outcomes. They would have to compete effectively on a playing field where general surgeons had been dominant for over a century.

From Subordinate Diagnosticians to Craft Challengers

Gastroenterological endoscopists responded to such criticism aggressively. Rather than delegate endoscopy to a marginal role in clinical medicine, they moved boldly toward operative therapy. For example, acknowledging the failure of diagnostic endoscopy to improve treatment outcomes for upper gastrointestinal bleeding, one commentator concluded that sending patients with "visible vessels" to surgeons might not be the best way to go. Instead of surgical treatment, he championed operative endoscopic modalities that were in experimental stages at the time, modalities capable of delivering treatment through the scope itself (NEJM 1979a). An interdisciplinary panel concluded in 1984 that operative endoscopic techniques, if used as alternatives to open surgery, might decrease mortality rates significantly (JAMA 1985).

The shift to operative endoscopy did not entail a radical skill disruption for gastroenterologists trained in diagnostic endoscopy. The operative instrument was simply inserted at the scope's base through a separate built-in channel. Access, the key to any successful operative procedure, was already established with the previous passing of the scope to the tissue of interest. All that was required to treat tissue was to thread a fiber through the scope, then send the energy flow to tissue through the fiber with a triggering mechanism. Although such techniques did require new knowledge and skills, such as basic understanding of the energy source and its tissue interactions, my endoscopic informants did not define picking up this knowledge as troublesome. As stated by a young gastroenterologist, "If you know endoscopy, then once you have, you know, you can learn in a day or two basic things. You can go and see the equipment. Give you some feel. You can find some animal experimentation lab and say, 'Let me do it.' . . . If you are good at endoscopic technique, and you understand tissue effects of laser, it should not be difficult."

The critical skills in operative endoscopy lie in passing the scope and interpreting tissue. These skills are the same whether endoscopists merely examine and diagnose tissue, or examine, diagnose, and treat it. The shift from diagnostic to operative procedures was defined in gastroenterological commentary as a natural development:

> Because the fiberoptic endoscope has placed the physician so tantalizingly close to the pathological processes with which he is dealing, attempts to deliver endoscopic therapy are the most natural outgrowth. One of the most promising of the many endoscopic therapeutic modalities is laser therapy. The appeal is broad based. The technique is relatively simple. The treatment does not involve tissue contact. The applications are potentially multiple. (AJG 1984c, 406; see also AJG 1978a, 534)

The shift to operative applications began rather innocently. First, small snares and baskets were threaded through the gastroscope to remove foreign objects accidentally swallowed. These techniques spared patients—mostly children—from invasive surgery (NEJM 1974). In the early 1970s gastroscopists began passing electrocautery probes through their scopes that allowed them to deliver electric current to tissue. They used these probes effectively to stop bleeding

(JAMA 1974a). Pioneering colonoscopists began to remove polyps in the colon, first with snares and electrocautery probes, later with lasers (see, for example, AJS 1978; JAMA 1974b; Lancet 1989; NEJM 1973c). Success with these early experimental techniques led to more ambitious approaches, including alternatives for stomach surgery and palliative cancer treatments (AJS 1988c; DCR 1993a; Gas 1985b). Complex nonsurgical endoscopic techniques for removing stones left in the biliary tract after surgery were also developed. These techniques were especially threatening to surgeons' claims regarding the superiority of surgical treatment (AJS 1988b; BMB 1986a; JAMA 1976b, 1977a; NEJM 1975, 1977d; 1992a). As the 1980s progressed, the endoscope's reach within the gastrointestinal tract grew wider and deeper. And, whenever the scope reached new terrain, it seemed that ambitious endoscopists were soon inventing ways to deliver treatment there.

Buoyed by their successes in first diagnostic and then operative endoscopy, some gastroenterologists began to question the legitimacy of the scripts that had long regulated workflow in the traditional division of labor between internal medicine and surgery. Developments in operative endoscopy challenged two fundamental assumptions of the normative order legitimated by these normative scripts.

First, these developments challenged the necessity of creating a division of labor between those specializing in diagnosis and those specializing in operative treatment. Such a division of labor was necessary when open surgery held superiority as the ultimate treatment alternative. Although surgical diagnosis might have been the more definitive approach, its costs to the vast majority of patients suffering from gastrointestinal conditions were severe. Screening medical from surgical conditions before an open incision was made became absolutely necessary.

Unlike the situation with open surgery, diagnosis and treatment are best combined during endoscopy in one time-bound performance. When endoscopists began to access tissue directly to diagnose conditions, adding a treatment function through the scope seemed natural and sensible. With blades, heater probes, electrocautery, or lasers, endoscopists learned that they could, on the spot, easily and effectively evaporate or excise the diseased or troublesome tissues they diagnosed. Although beneficial to patients, this unanticipated technological development challenged one of the foundational pillars of the normative order regulating workflow between internists and surgeons. Hence, the division of labor between diagnosis and operative treatment, and the specialization of work roles it had long entailed, suddenly stopped making sense. With the growing success of their own operative procedures, gastroenterological endoscopists increasingly refused to respect this division and its normative justification. They crossed the line to operative therapy and felt justified in doing so.

Second, the patient outcomes produced by endoscopic treatment were as measurable as were the outcomes produced by open surgery. Although some argued early on that the complication rates associated with endoscopy were too high for it to be used as a presurgical diagnostic exam, when it was used as an alternative method for treating tissue, its rates proved in many cases to be superior to those achieved in surgery. The complication rate for removing polyps from the colon through the endoscope, for example, was reported to be 23.3 per 1,000 in a 1975 survey conducted by the American Society of Gastrointestinal Endoscopy. This compared to a complication rate in open surgery of about 20 percent (JAMA 1975c). Because the procedure was less invasive, endoscopists argued that their technique should be preferred, as expressed in the following surgical commentary:

> Thinking of endoscopy simply as a new and more convenient way of performing surgery adds a fresh perspective to the debate (and reduces its heat). If we can show endoscopic therapy to be as effective and safe as orthodox surgery—not necessarily more so—then it must be preferred, since it is easier, quicker, cheaper, and produces less morbidity. The onus thus falls on the proponents of orthodox surgery to prove that the more invasive, expensive, and painful methods are more effective. (NEJM 1992b, 1627; see also JAMA 1981a)

A key pillar in the normative order favoring surgeons' dominance in the medical profession's division of labor was the measured and calculable superiority of surgical treatment over other treatment alternatives. Surgeons had relied on the meticulously documented outcomes of the beneficial effects of their surgical procedures throughout modern history. Such documentation was necessary to legitimate procedures that produced considerable trauma and hardships for patients. When the endoscopists began to challenge the efficacy of surgical treatment with the same empiricist logic that surgeons themselves had long embraced, surgeons were powerless to defend their own favored techniques, or to counter this logic with a viable alternative. The impressive documented outcomes of operative endoscopy legitimated gastroenterologists' program to extend their work jurisdiction across the time-honored demarcation line between medicine and surgery.

Once the normative legitimation of this demarcation line had become delegitimated by endoscopy's "natural" development, surgeons' markets became vulnerable because of their disadvantaged structural position. Simply put, gastroenterologists worked upstream in this division of labor; surgeons worked downstream. Patients with digestive problems generally were referred to the gastroenterologist before they ever saw the surgeon. And the referring physician was often a general internist who shared much of the same training and cultural orientation as the gastroenterologist. Because of this, gastroenterologists had first crack at influencing treatment choices. What the surgeon thought about what the gastroenterologist proposed was not of much consequence. However, the reverse did not hold. As a gastroenterological endoscopist I interviewed put it: "Interestingly for us, most of our referrals come from internal medicine or family physicians. Most of the surgery is generally not sent to the surgeons, unless they have gone to the gastroenterologist. . . . We have more say in these things."

Workplace environments are complex entities. No one can predict with certainty how these environments will respond to the demands of new technology. New technologies, with complexities of their own, often develop along trajectories that are unanticipated. Even when they are introduced into workplace environments in a manner respecting the existing normative orders regulating them, new technologies can develop in ways that might subsequently prove problematic. They may challenge the viability of the normative orders from which they originally drew support.

The case of fiber-optic endoscopy in gastrointestinal medicine is a case in point. This technology was introduced as a diagnostic tool. As such, the normative scripts regulating workflow legitimated the gastroenterologists' jurisdiction over the technology. At the time of the technology's introduction, gastroenterologists served in this division of labor as its master diagnosticians. Their primary role was to serve as consultants to primary care physicians in diagnosing their more difficult gastrointestinal cases. It seemed only natural and right that, as diagnosticians, the gastroenterologists should develop and control this technology. The general surgeons, in fact, conceded this early on, showing very little interest in the technology. Their interests and commitments were wedded to their operating room performances. Thus, fiber-optic endoscopy's initial course of development moved along a time-honored and legitimated path, a path well documented in the occupations and professions literature. This path was not challenging to the powers that be nor to the multiple interests that were served by the normative scripts regulating this division of labor.

That such a technology could turn so easily down a system-threatening path illustrates the potential vulnerability of this type of division of labor. The normative order regulating workflow in gastrointestinal medicine could not adapt itself well to the shift from diagnostic to operative endoscopic applications. And this shift was rather serendipitous—certainly not the result in its early stages of any master design for turf acquisition. By placing endoscopists' eyes so close to the tissue of interest, it seemed only natural that they would try to invent methods for treating it there. These efforts began simply as endoscopists threaded blades and loops through their scopes to accomplish simple operative tasks. As these efforts proved successful, they encouraged more ambitious efforts. And, with each success, the scripts regulating workflow in this division of labor lost a bit more of their common-sensical appeal and ultimately their legitimacy.

The challenge as to the ultimate value of diagnostic endoscopy actually functioned to hasten the transition from diagnostic to operative endoscopy. This challenge ultimately hurt those with a vested interest in preserving the existing normative order regulating the division of labor. For, rather than back away from their commitment to endoscopy, gastroenterologists began to question the efficacy of the surgeon's place in the division of labor when their own core virtue—accurate diagnosis—was challenged. Ambitious gastroenterologists, standing as outsiders to the surgeons' culture, increasingly came to believe that they could realize the full benefits of endoscopy only if they effectively challenged surgeons' dominance over treatment. Wherever possible, they attempted to develop endoscopic alternatives to open surgeries. When ambitious endoscopists successfully challenged surgery's dominance over ultimate treatments for gastrointestinal disorders with these alternatives, the hold of the normative scripts regulating this division of labor weakened considerably.

Whether we look at the advent of operative endoscopy as a natural outgrowth of the technology's development, as a defensive reaction to challenges to the technique's value as a diagnostic tool, or as a calculated power grab by ambitious young gastroenterologists operating within an increasingly glutted labor market—and a case can be made for all three—the ultimate consequence of this development was increasing turf conflict between medical and surgical practitioners treating digestive disorders. Whereas many entered the heat of this battle in partisan fervor, others lamented the deterioration of the cordial relations that once existed between the specialties. To understand this development more fully, we must turn to the peculiar set of labor-market dynamics structuring the occupational division of labor in medicine during the 1970s and 1980s.

6

State Mediation and Intraoccupational Developments

Scholars have long recognized that the state plays a critical role in shaping professional relationships. In fact, pure professionalism—where the occupation unilaterally dominates the relationships its practitioners establish with clients—is the exception in Terence Johnson's influential typology; other forms of control are thought to gain prominence as societies develop. Johnson (1972, chap. 6) discusses the particular case of state mediation as one of these. In state mediation the government becomes a direct, third-party player regulating the professional relationship. The practitioner–client relationship in U.S. medicine has shifted from a purer form of professionalism toward state mediation in the post–World War II period, beginning with the transition to state-sponsored research in the early years and intensifying during the 1960s and 1970s with the enactment of federal programs designed to increase the physician labor supply and with health insurance programs that involved the state directly in supplying, financing, and regulating services. This shift has had a number of consequences for occupational development, such as increasing the status and power of a research-oriented academic elite (Johnson 1972, chap. 6; see also Freidson 1984; Hoffman 1989, 39–40; Jamous and Peloille 1970, part 2; Marsden 1977, 81–83), encouraging occupational specialization and fragmentation (see Freidson 1984; Johnson 1972, chap. 6; Marsden 1977), and reducing practitioners' dependence on local referral networks (Freidson 1970b, 93–95; Galaskiewicz 1985; Shortell 1973, 4), among others.

Our concern is with documenting the impact of state mediation on the relationship between surgeons and gastroenterologists competing in the medical profession's internal division of labor. State mediation functioned to undermine surgery's leadership position at the same time that it increased competitive pressures in physician labor markets. These developments structured the terrain on which medicine and surgery battled for turf jurisdiction during the 1980s and 1990s.

Federal Policy and Medical Research

Until World War II organized medicine kept its core research, teaching, and clinical functions under its own unilateral control, integrating each function into the medical model outlined in the Flexner Report of 1910. The AMA defined the solo practitioner in fee-for-service practice as its ideal, and it resisted influences that might adversely affect the viability of this relationship, including state funding. Medical schools and residency programs defined the training of physicians for fee-for-service practice as their primary function. Research was tightly linked to the practical problems such practitioners experienced. Researchers supported their investigations primarily with grants from private-sector foundations. As late as 1940 the federal government funded less than 7 percent of medical research conducted in the United States (Hollingsworth 1986, 222–23).

Although Congress established a national institute of health in 1930, its budget and influence were meager. The model for more massive government involvement in medical research was set by the National Cancer Act of 1937 and the National Cancer Institute it created. This act singled out a specific disease for investigation and provided grants and training fellowships to independent researchers affiliated with both public and private institutions (Hollingsworth 1986, 223–24). In 1950 the Surgeon General established separate research institutes, referred to as the National Institutes of Health (NIH), to support investigations into a variety of specific diseases and disorders. Federal monies for research projects, and later for research fellowships, were granted to principal investigators through each of the fourteen major institutes of the NIH (Hollingsworth 1986, 224). The percentage of all biomedical research supported by the federal government increased from slightly less than 7 percent in 1940 to 45 percent in 1950 to over 60 percent in the mid-1960s through the mid-1970s (Hollingsworth 1986, 227; see also Stevens 1971, 358–60). As J. Rogers Hollingsworth (1986, 224) argues, the NIH effectively nationalized medical research.

The increased federal subsidies granted for medical research met little organized resistance from within the field of medicine. In the 1940s and 1950s the American Association of Medical Colleges (AAMC), claiming that the major medical schools it represented were in serious financial distress, actively sought support from the state. When bills proposing to subsidize medical school expenditures in exchange for increased enrollments all failed in Congress during the 1940s and 1950s, medical colleges and universities aggressively turned to NIH research grants and fellowships as a means of alleviating their financial plight. From the mid-1950s through the mid-1970s, over a third of the revenue coming to medical schools was from research grants, with the bulk of this underwritten by the federal government (Stevens 1971, 358–60; see also Feldstein 1977, 219).

Medical schools did not face strong opposition in increasing their dependence on federal research support. The AMA, although adamantly opposed to direct federal funding of medical schools, did not oppose research support (Stevens 1971, 351–52). The NIH were not threatening to the occupation's control over its labor supply because they did not fund medical school enrollments. Indeed, even with federal research grants flowing to medical schools, physician supply per population did not increase substantially during the 1950s. The AMA, aware of medical schools' financial difficulties, probably viewed the NIH as an acceptable alternative to direct subsidization and the specter of government regulation it threatened to bring about.

Nonetheless, federal support for medical research did have significant effects on the balance of forces in the medical profession's intraoccupational division of labor. Hollingsworth, among others, notes that massive federal research expenditures led to increases in occupational specialization and fragmentation, and even to the eventual breakdown of occupational solidarity and control (Hollingsworth 1986, 227–29; see also Fein and Weber 1971, 60; Light 1986). The NIH produced these results through the largely unintended and unanticipated effects of their grant systems on medical schools and residency programs.

The NIH allocated research funds to individual investigators, not to medical schools themselves, thus making researchers independent of institutional support from their home base. This significantly broke the power of medical school deans and department heads, weakening their capacities for uniting the profession, and/or its specialty segments, behind unified occupational programs. Rosemary Stevens (1971, 359–60) describes the newly decentralized structure of academic medicine as a system of "feudal baronies." And, as a result of NIH support, the ranks within these baronies increased threefold from 1962 to 1976 (Hollingsworth 1986, 229).

Our concern here is with the impact of these developments on the position of general surgery and gastroenterology in the medical profession's internal division of labor. Surgery, holding the dominant position during the early postwar period, had difficulty adapting to the changes engendered by state-sponsored expansion of the medical-research complex. Surgery's culture, and the action orientations it encouraged, was not ideally suited for taking advantage of the opportunities created by this expansion. Surgery's self-defined core virtues did not translate easily into the "pure science" model favored by the NIH. Surgery's position in the medical school power structure, and its ultimate place in the medical profession's internal division of labor generally, weakened as a result. Gastroenterology, on the other hand, a relatively new subspecialty of internal medicine that was hungry for status and power, saw the growth of the medical-research complex as an opportunity to advance its position within the division of labor. It reacted accordingly.

Surgery's Response

A strong clinical orientation had long dominated medical training in the United States, especially in surgery (see Becker et al. 1961; Bosk 1979). In the early 1900s, under the Halsted system, surgical residents often spent eight to twelve years working in hospitals as assistants to attending surgeons. Here, residents worked much like the apprentices in traditional handicrafts. They were expected to attain handicraft proficiency in all facets of surgery during this prolonged training period (see AJS 1965a, 1976a; Surg 1989; see also

ArchS 1990b; Surg 1973a). Surgical residents competed fiercely with one another in pyramid systems that offered progressively fewer and fewer positions as candidates advanced through the system. Only the very best rose to the chief resident positions in hospitals associated with the most prestigious medical schools (AJS 1965a; Surg 1970; SGO 1993). Such systems created a meritocratic hierarchy, with the most successful competitors rising to top positions in medical schools and surgical associations.

Surgical research was not at all shunned in this early environment. Rather, research interests were pursued pragmatically to resolve the clinical problems of the day. Surgeons drew from the rapidly advancing branches of the medical sciences to develop techniques for avoiding shock, trauma, and wound infection (AnnS 1967, 304–305). This early generation's successes in applying scientific advances to these practical problems, and in expanding the range of surgical treatments available in the process, were instrumental in organized medicine's rise to professional dominance in the United States. The type of practical research orientation employed here is akin to that found in traditional craft-based industries prior to the institutionalization of formal science. Knowledge is conceived of as an aid to practice. It is appropriated for uses defined by the needs of the practitioner.

The postwar expansion of the medical-research complex that was spurred by massive federal investments radically transformed the medical-research environment. Research subordinated to the practical needs of the clinician gave way to a form of research closer to the pure science paradigm lauded by the NIH. Biochemistry and biophysics, rather than gross anatomy, physiology, and bacteriology, provided the concepts and methods that guided this research. The research aims here were more abstract than those of the earlier period. They concerned the theoretical understanding of disease processes, their measurement and control. Research scientists, primarily oriented toward publication and funded lavishly through externally sponsored grants, became the major players in academic medicine as a result of this transformation. Their brand of science encouraged the detachment of research from problems of clinical practice, for the ultimate end of this research program was to revolutionize existing practice. These sciences tended to favor the development of treatments that were pharmaceutically based over those that were anatomical. Surgery, with its distinctive craft base, was disadvantaged in this milieu (AnnS 1967; see also AnnS 1963b, 775), while the newer subspecialties of internal medicine, like gastroenterology, embraced this change as an opportunity for advancing their status (AJS 1980f, 721; on the general shift in research sciences in medicine, see Fox 1989, 202).

The type of research scientist favored by the rapidly expanding medical-research complex was not easily nurtured in the surgeons' culture. Residency training, because of the nature of surgery's handicraft requirements, was reserved primarily for the development of procedural competence. The following surgical commentary expresses the dilemma posed by research:

> I always held the heretical thought that a surgeon could think, could be self-sufficient in the practice of medicine and, if an academician, could make research a part of his daily existence. I was discouraged from these concepts and told to apply myself to the time-honored format of ascending clinical responsibilities embodied in the difficulty of permitted operative procedures allocated to given years in residency training. Laboratory research, I was told, was an activity with which a gentleman-surgeon might dally subsequent to his training, provided that he did not have to earn a living. There was no room for even a year of research activity in the residency ladder. (AJS 1981b, 245)

Even those who argued that surgery must embrace the pure science model were quick to note the difficulties surgeons would have in doing so. As an academic surgeon stated in commentary: "Few academic surgeons of today are surgical scientists. We appear to lack a facility with thoughtful logic [that] would permit us to assess objectively the validity and significance of repetitive intelligent observations. Many seemingly lack the ability to apply scientific methods of thought" (AJS 1981b, 245; see also AJS 1967, 725).

There was more to this than mere psychological deficiency, however. The particularistic and individualistic values long lauded in clinical medicine were embraced most strongly in surgery. The surgical old guard defined a research method that required them to devalue their hard-earned experiential knowledge, to gloss over case-based particularities in favor of the establishment of the central tendency, and to routinize and fetter clinical judgment with a priori protocols as something anathema to what surgery was about (see, for example, AJS 1980f; AnnS 1967, 1969; NEJM 1978a). Surgery's craft essence conflicted strongly with the positivist-experimental ethos of the new milieu. Surgery, long defined as a particularistic application of general principles to unique and complex cases, did not lend itself to the type of abstraction and quantification favored by "pure" science. Although the outcomes produced by surgeons were made quantifiable and open to peer review, the craft processes producing these outcomes were defined in the surgeons' culture as impervious to codification, precise quantitative measurement, and external control.

Surgery's traditional, craft-based approach to the establishment of treatment protocols was increasingly difficult to legitimate in a milieu that embraced pure theoretical science. Surgeons had grown accustomed to adopting their favored treatments, at best, on the basis of their own retrospective analyses of their results. At worst, they did so on the basis of their idiosyncratic beliefs, even hunches. Such a mode of decision making was denigrated within the burgeoning medical-research complex, an environment that encouraged quantitative testing guided by the strictures of population sampling theory. Such an environment encouraged researchers to bask in the aura of certainty and finality that such testing fostered.

Yet, there was a strong rationale undergirding the surgeons' particularistic approach. Although randomized population testing was embraced successfully in experimental studies in medicine to advance the development of treatment protocols, such an approach could not be readily embraced in surgery. The variable having the strongest effect in determining surgical results was the handicraft skill of the surgeon as it was applied to the case during an uncertain, in-the-moment performance. This variable could not lend itself to the type of quantifiably expressed precision and standardization demanded in the double-blind study. The application of surgical skill varied in fundamental ways from surgeon to surgeon, case to case, even moment to moment. It defied accurate measurement. And it was defined in the surgeons' culture as having an indeterminate, perhaps mysterious—even mystical—quality.

Consequently, a plethora of techniques and approaches were employed in surgery, and no definitive method for deciding upon their value and place could conform to the "one-best-way" mantra favored in the positivist academic milieu of the postwar era. This relativistic approach was accepted as a natural state of affairs by most surgeons (Surg 1980b; see also AnnS 1979; ArchS 1978d; Surg 1980a; SCNA 1982c). And surgical innovations were seldom, if ever, submitted to the scientific controls required for adequately and objectively "testing" their efficacy. Once individual surgeons became convinced of their skill in delivering results with a new technique, they argued that it would be unethical to assign patients to control groups when they believed that the new technique could better help them (AJS 1967; Halm and Gelijns 1991; JAMA 1975b; for counter arguments, see JAMA 1975a). Clinical surgeons, with their careers and reputations heavily invested in delivering patient outcomes on a case-by-case basis, could not readily sacrifice immediate treatment outcomes to the abstract demands of positivist science.

In part because of its handicraft base, and the occupational values this engendered, surgery lagged behind other specialties in taking advantage of the opportunities created by the burgeoning medical-research complex. Other medical specialties, better equipped and motivated to adapt to the demands of the pure science model, leap-frogged quickly to the front of the NIH's grant lines (AnnS 1969, 646). Of course, they were encouraged to do so by their affiliated institutions, institutions often in dire need of funds.

The clinical surgeon rapidly lost status and prestige in this new environment. The first casualty was the "triple-threat" surgeon who excelled in all facets of academic surgery—patient care, teaching, and research (Surg 1983b, 123; see also SGO 1993). Where the traditional surgical residency esteemed and developed such surgeons, the new environment encouraged a dichotomization between research and patient care (AJS 1980f, 721). The relationship between these segments became increasingly antagonistic, as the latter lost status. As expressed by a Scottish surgeon experiencing similar developments:

> In the distant past a surgeon was judged by, and his reputation based on, technical prowess. During the past 30 years or so surgery has veered in a scientific direction and reputations are now largely based on scientific contribution. . . . Academic surgery holds the reins of influence. Concurrently, the attitude that operative surgery is easy, routine, universally adequate and not a sufficient intellectual stimulus for intelligent men has been tacitly promoted. (BJS 1987b, 1190; see also AJS 1976a, 141; AnnS 1969; NEJM 1978b)

The clinical surgeons' sense of lost status was expressed early on in surgical commentaries (AJS 1966, 624). Over the decades this sentiment deepened and became increasingly embittered, as expressed in the following commentary, "For the better part of my career, I have been reviled as a plumber and technician, insulted by my medical colleagues as being a carpenter who cuts on the doted line, and been told by 'beings of superior intellect' what the diagnosis is and how I should deal with it" (AJS 1989b, 275; see also AJS 1974b, 659; 1988a, 644–46; 1990f, 274).

This status loss was also evidenced in surgery's declining influence in medical education. Changes in medical education followed the state-sponsored expansion of the medical-research complex. Instruction shifted from a structured curriculum featuring training in the basic medical sciences to a looser model featuring more elective choices and more opportunities for pursuing specialty training and research earlier in students' careers. Some administrators thought that this new curriculum was better attuned to the realities of post-war medicine. Western Reserve pioneered this alternative in the 1950s, and by the 1960s the new curriculum was posing a serious challenge to all medical schools (Surg 1968a, 577).

The reforms did not bode well for surgery's position. Surgery was deemphasized at the M.D. level, and the hours students spent in surgical training significantly declined (ArchS 1983, 1017). Some expressed the view that the basic surgical sciences—particularly anatomy—were losing ground to the other sciences such as biochemistry and pathophysiology. One commentary linked surgical anatomy's declining influence directly to medical schools' "preoccupation with cash-generated research" (AJS 1980d; see also Surg 1974).

The depths to which surgery's status position had fallen became apparent when administrators and faculty committees began to float proposals for removing surgical training from the curriculum altogether. Those doing so conceived of surgery's knowledge base as equivalent to a handicraft skill best taught in post-M.D. residencies only to those desiring to enter the craft. This definition seemed to reverse the status gains that surgery had won during the early decades of the twentieth century. That medical school administrators and faculty colleagues were willing to entertain such proposals seriously shocked many academic surgeons and caused them to become defensive (AnnS 1968, 615; 1969, 648–49; Surg 1983b, 123). Influence in medical school training is important to a specialty's position in the division of labor, because it is here where the specialty makes first contact with potential recruits. This initial contact is vitally important to downstream specialties dependent upon others for patient referrals, as the surgical specialties are, for it is here that future colleagues gain an understanding of the given specialty's position and function in health care delivery (AJS 1976a, 141; CJS 1994a).

Thus, the rapid investment of federal funds in medical research in the early postwar period upset rather quickly the balance of forces established in the medical profession's internal division of labor. State mediation, and the rise of the medical-research complex that it sponsored, contributed, if unintentionally, to academic surgery's status deflation (ArchS 1983, 1017). The operating-room clinician—the heroic figure in the surgeons' culture, a figure that once towered over the medical profession—was displaced in the new milieu by the detached scientist working in the laboratory to expand our knowledge of diseases and their causes. Surgery's status deflation negatively affected its capacity for defending time-honored turf from the aggressive competitors spawned in this new and increasingly alien milieu.

Gastroenterology's Response

Gastroenterology's response to the rise of the state-sponsored medical-research complex contrasts starkly with surgery's. This is quite understandable. Whereas surgery had held a dominant position in the division of labor, gastroenterology's status was not well established. Gastroenterology was a young and hungry subspecialty of internal medicine seeking to enhance its prestige. From its standpoint, active state involvement in medical research was not a threat but a welcomed opportunity. Unlike surgery, gastroenterology was not wedded to a particular treatment modality; it did not have a long handicraft tradition. Consequently, gastroenterology was freer to embrace the pure science model favored by the NIH. And it actively sought NIH grant and fellowship support.

Gastroenterology began the postwar period in rather modest circumstances. Gastroenterologists competed for research support with ten other specialties and subspecialties in the National Institute of Arthritis and Metabolic Diseases (NIAMD). NIAMD funded research on the variety of illnesses that did not garner enough support, in themselves, to be the subjects of separate research institutes (Gas 1969b). In the academic years 1956–57 to 1963–64, the amount of research funding distributed through NIAMD increased over 18 percent each year. This rate declined in the later 1960s, however, to only 5.7 percent annually (Gas 1969a).

NIAMD granted gastroenterology two positions on its advisory

council. Those serving in these positions lobbied hard to increase
support for gastroenterology's research and fellowship programs.
They claimed a severe shortage of basic scientists and clinical researchers. Such lobbying paid off early on. In 1957 NIAMD began to
offer fellowships earmarked specifically for research and academic
careers in gastroenterology (Gas 1969b, 95).

The declining availability of research funds during the 1960s, however, was alarming to gastroenterology's NIAMD representatives.
They defined NIAMD's funding levels as much too meager to support the services the nation required for treating its gastrointestinal
problems (Gas 1969a). To mobilize support and recognition for its occupational program, the American Gastroenterological Association,
along with NIAMD and the Digestive Diseases Foundation, organized in 1967 the first national conference on gastrointestinal disease in the United States—the "Conference on Digestive Diseases as
a National Problem." Representatives attended the conference from
industry, government, the military, science, and education. The president of AGA defined this event as a milestone for the subspecialty.
The conference's aim was to assess the magnitude of the nation's gastrointestinal problems, the state of development of gastroenterology's knowledge base, and the level of funding needed to advance
gastroenterology's knowledge base and to treat these problems. The
conference report asserted that digestive diseases were the leading
cause of hospitalization in the United States. Such diseases caused
more hospital stays than any other organ system disease, the second
most lost workdays, and the third most deaths. However, the report
also indicated that the knowledge base for treating digestive disorders was underdeveloped and that gastroenterology lacked the research support and the physicians it needed to treat such disorders
effectively (Gas 1970). A second such conference was held in the
1970s (AJG 1978b; Gas 1967b; see also Gas 1976b, 1993c).

Such public relations efforts paid off. The increase in NIH fellowships that followed, coupled with gastroenterology's own impressive
innovations in science and in the development of endoscopic technology, triggered tremendous growth in the number of physicians entering the subspecialty (Gas 1992a). There were fewer than six
hundred certified gastroenterologists in practice during the 1960s
(Gas 1985a). As late as 1966, the American Board of Internal Medicine certified only twenty gastroenterological candidates (Gas 1985a;
see also Gas 1981b, 1982). From 1972 to 1983, in contrast, 3,385 gastroenterologists were certified, three times more than the total cer-

tified in all years prior to 1972. From 1975 to 1985, the number of gastroenterologists per 100,000 population increased from 1.1 to 2.4 (Gas 1989b).

Although all subspecialties of internal medicine grew rapidly in response to the opportunities created by NIH grants and fellowships, gastroenterologists fared quite well in comparison to their internist colleagues. As a percent of the total pool of certified internists practicing in the United States, gastroenterologists increased from 4.2 percent in 1978 to 6.0 percent by 1990 (Gas 1985b; see also SCNA 1982e, 582). From 1965 to 1990, the number of certified gastroenterologists increased 1,083 percent, a rate of increase higher than that for cardiology (734 percent) (Gas 1993d).

Thus, gastroenterology, a field spawned largely by NIH grants and fellowships in the new medical-research complex, and popularized by its growing technological prowess, came of age in the 1980s as a powerful medical subspecialty. The enormous swelling of the gastroenterological ranks, however, set off expansionary impulses that quickly threatened to burst the specialty's jurisdiction well beyond its traditional line of demarcation. This, however, was hardly an afterthought to those leading gastroenterology's occupational program in the new state-sponsored, medical-research milieu.

Federal Policy and Physician Training

The federal government's impact on the medical profession soon extended well beyond the research function. In 1963 Congress passed a bill that directly subsidized medical school expansion in exchange for increased enrollments. This gave the state, for the first time, a direct mechanism for increasing the number of practicing physicians in the United States. And the state used this mechanism to break organized medicine's grip on its labor supply. Newly minted M.D.s flooded the market in the 1970s and 1980s, and, as noted in the literature, this spurred intense turf competition within and between specialties (see, for example, Ginzberg 1984; Ginzberg et al., 1981, 511–12, 525–26).

Policies and Outcomes

From the 1960s through the 1970s, the federal government took aggressive action to relieve an alleged physician shortage. Congress established the first federal subsidy program for medical schools with the Health Professions Educational Assistance Act of 1963 (PL 88-129). This act provided three-year support for construction funds to schools in exchange for one-time enrollment increases. The 1963 act also established the first federally supported loan program for medical students (Fein and Weber 1971, 199–201; Feldstein 1977, 62–65; Ginzberg 1986; 1990, 192–93; LeRoy and Lee 1977, 1–2, 216; Litman 1991, 402–403). The act was renewed in 1965 and 1968. It was expanded in 1971 as the Comprehensive Manpower Act (PL 92-157). The 1971 act provided per capita funds to medical schools in exchange for percentage increases in enrollments (see Altman 1984, 10–12; Lawton and Glisson 1984; LeRoy and Lee 1977, 3, 21; Litman 1991, 403).

In the 1980s, federal policy changed fundamentally. The Health Manpower Training Act of 1976 (PL94-184) actually declared an abrupt end to the alleged physician shortage. The 1976 act did continue capitation support to medical schools. However, such support was now contingent upon assurances that half of medical school graduates would pursue primary care careers. Direct capitation subsidies were eliminated altogether in 1981 (Litman 1991, 406). In 1986 the AMA House of Delegates forecast a severe physician surplus and called for corrective actions (Ginzberg 1990, 192–93).

The federal government's attempt to increase the supply of physicians in the 1960s and 1970s marked a substantial policy change. The AMA historically had defined government funding of medical school training as a direct threat to its control. It staunchly refused to support such policies after World War II. Even in the face of alleged physician shortages, the AMA claimed that a physician surplus existed during the late 1940s. And medical schools graduated the same number of physicians in 1949 as they did in 1940. The physician-per-population ratio for 1949 was 135 physicians per 100,000 population, a one-physician-per-100,000-population increase from the 1942 ratio. This ratio changed little throughout the 1950s, even in the face of studies that indicated a serious physician shortage, even in the face of mounting public pressure to train more physicians. Several bills were introduced in Congress during the 1940s and 1950s that aimed to grant federal aid to medical schools in exchange for increased enrollments. The AMA lobbied successfully to defeat each one (Stevens 1971, 353–58; see also Feldstein 1977, 62–63). In the early postwar years the AMA defined state funding as a precursor to a form of state regulation that would threaten the profession's control of its labor supply. As Stevens noted, "Implicit in governmental subsidy of medical education were questions of potential governmental control over an area which was at the core of the concept of professionalism: the freedom to describe, to choose, to regulate new entrants to the profession" (1971, 352).

However, the AAMC broke ranks with the AMA on this policy. Medical colleges and universities were beset by severe financial problems in the postwar period. Federal funds were readily available for hospital construction and for sponsored medical research, and medical schools quickly took advantage of these opportunities. However, these funds could not cover basic operating costs, and little funding was available for direct teaching support (Stevens 1971, 366–67). Many of the leading medical schools were forced to apply for distress grants from the federal government to make ends meet. Hence, the economic incentive for the medical schools that were represented by the AAMC to support such federal subsidies was quite transparent, as was the incentive for the AMA, and the established practitioners it represented, to oppose them.

A number of studies were commissioned during the period that forecast a severe physician shortage if medical school enrollments were not quickly expanded. And, left to itself, the medical profession did not look capable of or willing to increase physician supply. Indeed, as Stevens reported (1971, 365), the ratio of physicians per population actually fell during the decade spanning 1950 to 1960. In 1952 the President's Commission on the Health Needs of the Nation forecast a physician shortage of over 50,000 by the 1960s. The Surgeon General's Consultation Group on Medical Education published two very influential reports: the Bane-Jones Report in 1958, and the Bane Report in 1959. These reports predicted a need for 11,000 medical graduates per year until 1975 just to maintain the existing physician-per-population ratio, a ratio many defined as inadequate. This report noted the discrepancy between research and teaching in medical school budgets and recommended direct government aid to medical schools in order to rectify the problem (Stevens 1971, 362–63; see also Fein and Weber 1971, 196–97; Feldstein 1977, 62–65; LeRoy and Lee 1977, 22). The AAMC embraced wholeheartedly the recommendations made in these reports (Feldstein 1977, 64–65, 206; see also Fein and Weber 1971, 201).

These reports were used to champion the cause of the 1963 Health

Professions Education Assistance Act. The AMA had put itself in a difficult public-relations position and began to acknowledge the physician shortage that so many others were claiming. The AMA did not mobilize its resources to fight the passage of the 1963 act. It accepted the act's provision for one-time construction grants to medical schools. Eli Ginzberg (1986, 2–3) argued that the AMA leadership was preoccupied with mobilizing its resources to defeat the Medicare bill and, because of this, allowed the Health Professions Act to slip by without strong opposition. The AMA did oppose, however, federally supported student grants and fellowships. Paul Feldstein suggested that the AMA leadership saw this provision as a potential threat to its class and ethnic homogeneity (Feldstein 1977, 64–65). Whatever its motives, the AMA in 1968 joined with the AAMC to support the act's renewal (Ginzberg et al. 1981, 511–12). With the funds provided by these acts medical school construction increased substantially during the 1960s (Altman 1984, 10).

This infusion of state funds was not enough to relieve the medical schools' financial distress. Lauren LeRoy and Philip Lee (1977, 22) reported that the majority of medical schools applied for financial distress grants in 1970, including some of the most prestigious schools in the country. This condition was addressed in a new study sponsored by the Carnegie Commission. The 1970 Carnegie Commission Report forecast a severe physician shortage by 1975 and recognized the medical schools' severe financial problems and their inability to finance the increased enrollments needed to avert this. The Commission proposed capitation grants as the solution to both problems. The Commission requested that, in exchange for the increased revenue, medical schools increase enrollments 15,300 by 1976 and 16,400 by 1978 (Feldstein 1977, 228; see also Cooper and Olimpio 1980). The Comprehensive Manpower Act of 1971, in effect, implemented the Carnegie Commission's proposal. And the capitation grants provided did relieve medical schools' financial problems. Only a single school applied for financial distress grants two years after the act was passed (LeRoy and Lee 1977, 22).

As planned, direct capitation grants substantially increased the physician supply. From 1946 to 1963, before the government subsidies, the average annual rate of increase in medical school graduates was a quite modest 1.4 percent. This can be viewed as the occupation's own response to the growing concern over the projected physician shortage. From 1964 to 1971, after the passing of the first Health Professions Educational Assistance Act but prior to capitation grants, the average annual rate of increase rose to 2.7 percent. From 1972 to 1980, after capitation grants were enacted, the average annual rate jumped to 6.0 percent (percentages calculated from Wilsford 1991, table 4.2). In 1963, there were eighty-seven medical schools in the United States that enrolled 32,001 students and graduated 7,331. In 1975, there were 114 medical schools that enrolled 54,074 students and graduated 12,714. This constituted an increase in enrollments of 69 percent for the thirteen-year period (LeRoy and Lee 1977, 22; see also Altman 1984, 10; Cooper and Olimpio 1980, 36; Feldstein 1977, 203). The physician-per-100,000-population ratio also increased dramatically—from 136 in 1960 to 156 in 1970 to well over 200 in 1990 (figures from Light 1986, 519; the figure for 1990 is an estimate; see also Ginzberg 1984, 117). Of course, federal funding made this expansion possible. From 1969 to 1974, federal funds to medical education more than doubled (LeRoy and Lee 1977, 108–109).

The rapid expansion of the physician supply spurred by these capitation grants did not resolve problems of health care access for many Americans, however. The most important failure of this legislation, for our interests here, was the failure to address the impact of physician maldistribution by specialty and the influx of physicians trained in non-U.S. medical schools into U.S. residency programs. Both developments were outcomes of the enormous expansion of the medical-research complex in the postwar period discussed above. The number of M.D.s entering primary care specialties dropped substantially in the postwar period, as graduate fellowships became readily available from the NIH. LeRoy and Lee report that the physician-per-100,000-population ratio for primary care physicians had actually declined from 94 in 1931 to 55 in 1974 (LeRoy and Lee 1977, 145–46). Students entering medical training during the 1960s and 1970s continued to enter residencies, and then often subspecialty fellowships, after they obtained their M.D. degrees. Such specialization was encouraged by the expanding number of positions offered. Ginzberg reported that, as late as 1983, the total number of residency positions offered was greater than the total number of graduates from U.S. and non-U.S. schools applying for positions (Ginzberg 1984, 73). The problem with this was that both the number and type of graduate positions offered were generated not by a concern with future patient need but by a concern with what the NIH were currently willing to fund.

Beginning in the 1960s, hospitals and university medical centers

were turning to foreign medical graduates (FMGs) to fill labor shortages created by the state-sponsored research boom. In 1961, less than
6 percent of all physicians were FMGs. In 1967, 23 percent of newly
licensed physicians and 15 percent of all practitioners were FMGs.
By 1974, these numbers had grown to 40 percent and 21 percent re-
spectively (Altman 1984, 10–12; see also ArchS 1971b). In 1973, for
the first time, more FMGs entered the United States than there were
graduates from U.S. medical schools (Feldstein 1977, 67). Henry
Wechsler noted that almost one half of the gain made in total physician supply from 1960 to 1970 came from FMGs (Wechsler 1976,
124). The projections used in the 1971 Comprehensive Manpower
Act did not take into account the rapid influx of FMGs into the country to meet the growing labor demands of hospitals and university
medical centers. Where the 1970 Carnegie Report anticipated that
the needed 50,000-physician increase would be met by 1982 if its proposals were enacted, the projected target actually was exceeded after
only four years. Although the AMA opposed the rapid increase in the
number of FMGs, hospitals and attending physicians needed their labor to fill their residency and fellowship positions, and this labor was
subsidized by the state. Hospitals were reluctant to reduce their labor force by losing residents, as stated in the following commentaries: "No surgical staff or hospital administrator will willingly
reduce its number of residents by any significant figure, such as 25
to 30 percent. The trustees, administration, and attending staff of a
hospital disagree about many things. But they will agree on one
thing, if nothing else: recruit, attract, appoint, keep, and keep happy
the surgical residents" (Surg 1972, 661; see also Hiestand 1984, 71);
and "I have a feeling that it is the climate and needs within the training institutions and not the needs of society that presently dictate
the output of new gastroenterologists. Institutional staffs pressured
by teaching, research, and academic loads do not have the time to
handle personally the recent explosion of procedures without an
army-in-training to do them" (Gas 1978c, 1348). One commentator
linked the total number of residents in postgraduate training to a program's ability to receive and renew NIH grants (AJG 1983b, 58).

The federal government did take action to redress this problem in
the late 1970s and early 1980s. Congress passed an immigration law
in 1976 that restricted the number of FMGs entering residencies (Litman 1991, 405; see also SCNA 1982d, 608). Capitation grants were
eliminated in 1981; grant and loan support was reduced as well

(Ginzberg 1984, 118). Funds available to sponsored research also declined, and medical schools were forced to increasingly rely on funds from patient services to cover operating costs. The proportion of medical school budgets covered by such services increased considerably during the 1980s (Surg 1988, 116; see also Hiestand 1984, 50, 52; Surg 1983b, 122–23).

Surgery's Response

The labor-market transformations set in motion by federal policy did not favor surgery's position in either academia or in general practice. In the early 1970s surgeons mobilized their internal resources to develop a program to counter the impact of federal policies on their market position. Surgery's occupational program, more than that of any other specialty, anticipated early on the deleterious effects of state mediation and attempted to counter them. Surgery was more successful than its competitors in controlling its internal labor supply.

The American Surgical Association and the American College of Surgeons initiated in 1970 an unprecedented $1.5- million study of the surgical labor market—the "Study on Surgical Services in the United States" or SOSSUS. The reports it generated challenged prevailing assumptions regarding federal policy and its impact on the surgical labor supply (AnnS 1976; ArchS 1977; JAMA 1976c; NEJM 1976a, 1976b, 1981a, 1981d; Surg 1978b; see also Feldstein 1977, 206; LeRoy and Lee 1977, 148; Millman 1980, 16–17). SOSSUS can be read as an ambitious occupational program advanced by surgeons to regain control over their labor markets.

It is perhaps most prudent to report first what SOSSUS did not do. SOSSUS did not conclude that too many qualified surgeons were practicing surgery in the United States. Such a simplistic reading was soundly criticized in surgical commentary. SOSSUS actually concluded that the demand for surgical services in the United States could be meet sufficiently with the existing supply of board-certified surgeons (Millman 1980, 18; see also AJS 1986a). The problem disrupting this balance by the 1970s was the alarming number of physicians performing surgery without board certification. On the basis of its surveys, SOSSUS concluded that 92,000 physicians were performing surgeries in the United States in 1970. Only 50,000 of these were board certified, however, and only 12,000 of the remainder were residents on track to become certified. The rest were physicians without credentials in surgery—M.D.s who dropped out of surgical residencies or who had failed their credentialing examinations, as well as general practitioners performing minor procedures (see AJS 1981a, 634; Surg 1978b, 116; see also JAMA 1977d). This situation resulted historically from surgery's failure to establish full and formal monopolistic closure over its services. No laws were ever passed in the United States restricting the services a licensed medical doctor could offer patients, and many hospitals granted operating privileges without certification checks. In response to this, SOSSUS called for stricter hospital guidelines for granting surgical privileges and called upon the Joint Commission on Accreditation of Hospitals to enforce credentialing requirements (see Millman 1980, 18; Surg 1972, 1978b). Of course, this policy favored the market position of board-certified surgeons. It was designed to secure monopoly closure around their service markets (Surg 1978b, 118; see also Moore's commentary in ArchS 1974, 638).

A second problem that was threatening to disrupt the market balance SOSSUS sought was the influx of newly minted M.D.s flocking to surgical residencies in response to both the state-sponsored increases in medical school enrollments during the 1960s and the state-sponsored expansion of residency programs during the 1950s and 1960s. SOSSUS reported that from 1971 to 1975 the number of board-certified surgeons grew from 46,500 to 55,000, a growth rate reported to be seven times that of the general population (Surg 1978b, 116). And state policies that increased medical school enrollments at the time portended greater increases in surgeons' numbers in the future.

The solution advocated by SOSSUS was for surgery's own regulatory bodies to assert stricter control over the certification of internship and residency programs. SOSSUS legitimated this under the banner of quality control. One proposal would restrict expansion of surgical residencies to only a 1-percent increase in the surgeon-per-population ratio every five years. This proposal would protect surgical labor markets from surpluses in the future (AnnS 1976, 125–6; see also Surg 1978b, 116; SCNA 1982e, 598).

The survey questionnaires collected and analyzed by SOSSUS showed strong support from the surgical community for its recommendations. Of general surgeons surveyed, for example, 47 percent reported that they believed that there were too many general surgeons in practice, while only 3 percent reported that they believed a shortage existed (Surg 1977). Ninety-four percent supported a proposal for restricting surgical privileges to only those who were board certified or board eligible. Eighty-four percent supported a proposal that would require those without credentials to pass equivalency certification (Surg 1976, 631).

Surgery's gatekeepers acted quickly and effectively to put the SOS-SUS recommendations into effect. General surgery decreased the number of its weakest residency programs—those unaffiliated with medical schools—by 75 percent from 1970 to 1978 (AJS 1986a, 571). Although the number of surgeons in practice grew from 1970 to 1980, general surgery's growth rate was much slower than that of other medical and surgical specialties (AJS 1986a; SCNA 1982e, 581). The number of residents entering surgical programs declined significantly after the publication of the SOSSUS reports. The total number of M.D.s entering residencies in surgery and surgical specialties dropped from 1,848 in 1973–74 to 1,597 in 1980–81, a 14-percent drop. The number entering general surgery residencies dropped from 482 in 1973–74 to 352 in 1980–81, a 34 percent drop (SCNA 1982d, 607–608). In response to a number of factors, the number of surgical residents stabilized in the 1980s. The percent of medical students intending to enter surgery dropped from the historic level of one-quarter to one-third of all those planning to enter residency training to a low mark of 13 to 14 percent in the 1980s (ArchS 1983, 1017; Surg 1989; SCNA 1982d). The Council on Graduate Medical Education (COBRA) presented its report on the physician labor supply to Congress in 1988. COBRA concluded that, although there was generally an oversupply of physicians that would intensify in the near future, demand for surgeons would soon exceed supply. The massive glut of surgeons predicted in the 1970s did not fully materialize, largely because of the occupational program instituted by surgery's gatekeepers (ArchS 1983). However, by the 1970s, surgery's internal discipline and control was no longer sufficient to influence the behavior of the other medical specialties competing for dominance and markets.

Gastroenterology's Response

Unlike general surgery, gastroenterology did not attempt to restrict the growth of its labor supply in response to forecasts of a physician oversupply during the 1980s. As a relatively new subspecialty, gastroenterology initially had welcomed the opportunities for growth made possible by government subsidies. In the 1960s and 1970s gastroenterology needed to attract committed recruits to its fellowship programs in order to advance its status position. It welcomed new recruits, and this policy died hard. Gastroenterology's governing bodies make no major attempt to study and forecast the gastroenterological labor market, apart from participating in the general studies reporting on the general state of the nation's physician supply (Gas 1978b; 1981a, 861).

Nevertheless, by the 1980s clinical gastroenterologists felt keenly the threat of a saturated labor market. Numerous commentaries were published expressing concern over the burgeoning numbers of M.D.s flocking to gastroenterological fellowship programs, the intensifying competition, and the potential for skill dilution in the face of dwindling case loads (Gas 1978a, 1978b, 1978c). Seventy-two percent of the gastroenterologists reported in a 1986 American College of Gastroenterology (ACG) membership survey that they expected to experience increased competition in the future. Increasing competition was also identified as one of the top problems facing gastroenterology during the 1980s and 1990s (AJG 1987e, 1008).

Yet the market pressure experienced by gastroenterologists was very different from that felt by general surgeons. General surgeons in community practice began to experience the fallout of an oversupply in the early 1970s, while gastroenterologists began to experience the same thing a decade or so later. Most importantly, general surgeons offered services that had limited market appeal. Because of their specialty's maturity and its high level of technical sophistication and development, it was unlikely that abdominal surgeons would discover new, market-expanding applications for treating abdominal conditions. As a consequence, general surgery's market boundaries were fixed and rather rigid. Gastroenterologists, on the other hand, had opportunities opening to them for expanding their market turf during the 1980s and 1990s, as endoscopy shifted from diagnostic to treatment applications.

Indeed, some gastroenterological commentary questioned the validity of reports forecasting an oversupply of trained gastroenterologists. They argued forcefully that gastroenterology's impressive technological developments—particularly in endoscopy—would pave the way for new applications that would expand the service market for the growing legions of physicians entering gastroenterological training (AJG 1987b; 1987d, 881; 1989). That these new opportunities would have to come at the expense of general surgery did not seem a pressing concern to those advocating such a position. By the 1980s the subdisciplines of internal medicine no longer respected the line of demarcation that once existed between medical and surgical treatments. Internal medicine—particularly gastroenterology—was poised to invade time-honored surgical turf.

The most profound consequences of the federal government's policies, for our interests, were those that were unintended and perhaps unanticipated—those that, when coupled with the impact of the rise of the state-supported medical-research complex, profoundly disrupted the balance of forces operating within medicine's internal division of labor. The increasing number of newly minted M.D.s graduating from state-subsidized medical schools in the 1960s and 1970s quickly entered residency and fellowship programs, subsidized largely by federal research grants. This rapidly expanding supply of highly specialized physicians, coupled with a finite demand in the population for the services that they were trained to deliver, created intense, unprecedented labor-market pressure. This pressure intensified competition and rivalry between specialties serving similar markets. It intensified competition greatly between medicine and surgical specialties sharing organ or disease systems generally; it intensified the competition between gastroenterologists and general surgeons in particular. By the 1980s, general surgeons no longer had the moral authority within the occupation to regulate destructive competition. Within this unprecedented labor-market context, the embrace of the new technology took on a rather peculiar and, at times, desperate form.

7

Turf Wars over the
Gastrointestinal Tract

Service markets regulated by professionalism, in theory, do not follow the simple logic of supply and demand forces. Professionals, because they are in a position to define client needs, can respond to increases in their labor supply by simply increasing client demand for the services that they perform. Although we hope that professionals' commitment to their ethical code will moderate such self-interest, the control structures operating within professions like medicine are generally much too weak to force the issue. And, indeed, general surgeons in the United States, apparently in response to the state-mandated increase in their labor supply, initially did increase the number of operations they performed. From 1966 to 1978 this number increased by 26 percent (Surg 1981c, 151). Such an increase, in the absence of other apparently compelling forces, led observers to suggest that a kind of Parkinson's Law operated in surgery, such that the number of operations performed would simply increase concomitantly with increases in the number of surgeons working in an established market (McPherson et al. 1981; see also Hollingsworth 1986, 108; Wechsler 1976, 128–29). This prospect alarmed the public, the press, and ultimately the profession, as it suggested that something other than concern for patients was motivating surgical decision making. The prospects of economically motivated "unnecessary surgery" received scathing criticism in the press. This further tarnished the reputation of surgeons and produced concern, anxiety, defensiveness.

By the 1980s, however, the alarm over increasing surgical rates proved unwarranted. Surgical rates leveled off in the later 1970s, even as the supply of surgeons continued to grow (AJS 1974b; SCNA 1982b; see also ArchS 1983, 1017). In the early 1980s the number of operations performed per surgeon actually decreased by 25 percent. The surgical market contracted notably during the 1980s (BMB 1986d, 221–22; Chang and Luft 1991, 112; JAMA 1980b; Lancet 1993c; NEJM 1982a; Wilsford 1991, 17).[1] Whatever power surgeons may have once had to influence the demand for their services had all but vanished. This power was taken away, not by a consumer revolt, nor by an alarmed and vigilant free press, nor even by a powerful state or third-party regulator—although it can be argued that each had its own modest influence. Rather, the primary forces responsible for the decline in surgical markets in the United States were aggressive competitors from within the medical profession, who offered patients attractive and viable treatment alternatives.

In response to their turf losses to these competitors general surgeons eventually were forced to change their orientation to the scope technology. To protect their livelihoods in an increasingly uncertain environment surgeons embraced the gastrointestinal endoscope during the 1980s and staked claims over its operative applications. However, the market outcomes of this belated attempt to incorporate endoscopy into the surgical armamentarium were only modest at best. Surgeons, by and large, could not wedge their way into the endoscopic markets that the gastroenterologists had already developed.

Assault on Surgical Markets

In the 1970s about a quarter of the time and effort that general surgeons spent in the operating room was expended on three major operations: gallbladder removals, hernia repairs, and appendectomies. These were considered the general surgeons' bread-and-butter operations. Surgeons performed them regularly; they honed their skill and efficacy on them; and they defined these operations as the core procedures through which they demonstrated their occupational virtue. Although these core procedures held central position in the definitional frame of general surgery, most of surgeons' operating-room time and effort was spent performing dozens of other intra-abdominal procedures (ArchS 1978c). Each of these was performed less frequently than the bread-and-butter procedures, but, taken together, they constituted the bulk of general surgeons' operating load.

Many of these latter procedures were challenged and often replaced during the 1980s by pharmaceutical, radiographic, and/or endoscopic treatments. These alternatives either replaced open surgeries completely, or they reduced their incidence to the rare, special-status case. These alternatives effectively removed the surgeon from the medical team that evaluated, diagnosed, and treated patients with such conditions. Holding the downstream position in health care delivery, and having much of their authority deflated during the period in question, general surgeons were powerless to reverse this course.

Drugs have historically competed with surgery in treating illnesses. And one of the consequences of the massive investment in biomedical research in the postwar period was the development and improvement of pharmaceutical treatments for a host of conditions once defined as surgical. For general surgeons, one of the most significant of these was Glaxo's Zantac, a medication that first became available for treating gastric ulcers in the 1980s, and which was followed shortly thereafter by a plethora of similar medications (AJS 1986b, 15; Chang and Luft 1991; CJS 1993a; Wilsford 1991, 17). Such medications were designed to correct the chemical imbalances within the gastrointestinal tract that eventually caused stomach and intestinal ulcers. In the past, the most serious of these had to be treated surgically. Stomach operations constituted a significant component of surgeons' workload.

Pharmaceutical treatments gained general favor over surgeries during the period of focus here. Such treatments, however, are not always better for patients. When the cause of a given illness lies in anatomical conditions that can be corrected effectively with surgical reconstruction, and when such surgery has a reasonably low risk of morbidity and a negligible risk of mortality, then surgery spares patients the costs and the side effects associated with taking toxic medications over an extended period. In the past, the medical profession accepted this logic and readily referred patients with such conditions to surgeons.

However, once this logic began to loose sway, surgeons were not in strong position to argue effectively in defense of their treatments, since they worked downstream in a dependent position within the health care delivery system. Internists, working upstream, were in a position to make moot the surgeons' arguments. When internists refused to offer the surgical alternative to patients, or if they chose to try the medical treatment first, perhaps defining it as the less invasive of the choices available, patients were not given access to general surgeons' opinions on their treatment courses. This made surgical markets quite vulnerable to the development of pharmaceutical treatments, particularly as surgery's status position had fallen within medicine. Surgical markets were assaulted frequently during the 1980s as new pharmaceutical treatments were developed and marketed heavily to primary care physicians.

Radiologists constituted another market threat. Aside from the major operations involving organ removals or significant anatomical reconstruction, general surgeons traditionally had performed a host of lesser surgical procedures that were palliative or diagnostic in nature, such as draining adhesions or taking tissue biopsies. Many of these were taken over in the 1970s and 1980s by radiologists who discovered that, with the aid of fluoroscopic techniques, they could locate precisely the organ or tissue of interest and access it effectively by merely inserting needles through the skin. This type of procedure was sufficient for draining pus, for taking small tissue samples, and later for shrinking and removing tissue through small punctures with electrical current. Such techniques made open surgeries unnecessary. Although immensely beneficial to patients, such procedures no doubt contributed to the reduction of general surgeons' workloads. They enabled radiologists to complement developments in endoscopic gastroenterology and, at times, to compete with gastroenterologists for market turf that was once monopolized by the surgical craft (AJG 1990; AJS 1988a, 5; ArchS 1991d, 1176; SCNA 1982e, 585).

Perhaps the biggest threat to general surgeons' secondary procedures during the 1980s was the gastrointestinal endoscope. As discussed earlier, the endoscope was used by enterprising gastroenterologists and a few surgeons early on to stop bleeding sources in the gastrointestinal tract and to remove polyps from the colon, procedures that once were performed surgically. In the 1980s the sophistication and the range of operative endoscopy increased, and this challenged surgeons' grip on their markets.

One of the most impressive developments was endoscopic retrograde cholangiopancreatography (ERCP). This method initially enabled gastroenterologists to obtain reliable images of the pancreatic and ductal systems prior to surgery, to pinpoint more precisely the nature of the gastrointestinal disorder afflicting the patient, and to avoid unnecessary incisions and puncture wounds (see, for example, AJG 1977, 1988b; AnnS 1986a). Gastroenterologists and some radiologists then developed methods to treat conditions endoscopically within the biliary tract by inserting instruments either percutaneously or through the endoscope. For example, endoscopists began inserting catheters through the scope to drain bile that was blocked by inflamed tissue in the pancreatic-biliary system. They also developed procedures for stenting obstructed pathways, as well as for inserting feeding tubes through the scope (see, for example, AJG 1978c, 1984b, 1984d, 1986c). All of these procedures required open surgery prior to this development. With endoscopy, patient management of these conditions shifted from the surgeon to the internist.

In time, gastroenterologists developed endoscopic methods for breaking up and removing stones lodged in the biliary tract. This development was especially threatening to surgeons, who generally had refused to adopt intraoperative endoscopic techniques for diagnosing and removing such stones (AJS 1980e, 7; 1988a, 5; CJS 1993a). Not only did this development pass another market to nonsurgeons, perhaps more importantly, it challenged the viability and superiority of a time-honored surgical treatment. The treatment outcomes of stone removal with ERCP were far superior to those of open surgery. The endoscopic technique for removing common bile duct stones sported a morbidity rate of approximately 10 percent and a mortality rate of less than 1 percent. The open surgical technique, in contrast, sported a mortality rate of approximately 10 percent for patients over sixty-five (AJG 1986a; see also AJG 1978c, 1984b, 1988a, 1272).

Surgeons, who had legitimated their own procedures by the measurable treatment results they produced, were forced to accept the validity of the ERCP operative alternatives. They did attempt to delimit the use and extension of these alternatives, however, by drawing a firm line of demarcation between surgical and endoscopic turf. Surgeons argued that such treatments should be used routinely for removing common bile duct stones only after surgeons removed the gallbladder through the traditional open technique, and only after they performed intraoperative cholangiography to locate and remove the most accessible stones lodged in the biliary tract (ArchS 1979; see also ArchS 1994b–e). Regardless of the objective merits of this argument, its acceptance left the management of the gallbladder case firmly in the surgeons' hands. Under the sway of this argument, the incidence with which surgeons performed their bread-and-better gallbladder procedure did not change, and surgeons had first option of locating and removing stones intraoperatively. Under this argument's sway, surgeons lost only their postsurgical procedures to the gastroenterological endoscopists. Although perhaps begrudgingly, they did learn to accept the endoscope's place in gallstone treatment as an adjunct to open surgery.

However, by 1990 the sway of this compromise argument had weakened. Gastroenterologists, emboldened by their endoscopic successes, began to challenge the general surgeons' time-honored control over the management of the traditional gallbladder case. One gastroenterological commentary argued that, given their success rates, endoscopic approaches to stone management should be used prior to open gallbladder removal, in some cases sparing patients from surgery altogether (AJG 1988a). One surgical commentator confirms that such a movement was afoot within the gastroenterological community in the 1990s, a movement that would have minimized further the general surgeons' role in the management of gallbladder cases (ArchS 1994d). New nonsurgical techniques were also being developed at this time for managing gallstone diseases. These experimental techniques promised to restrict surgical markets even further. At this point, internal medicine's assault on surgical markets appeared to many increasingly desperate general surgeons to be beyond containment.

General Surgery Embraces the Scope

As discussed in chapter 4, general surgery's initial response to the fiber-optic endoscope was consistent with the normative expectations that had evolved over the years within the medical profession's internal division of labor. Surgery, a treatment-oriented specialty, delegated the scope's development to internal medicine, inasmuch as the scope's primary application was thought to be diagnostic at the time. This strategy was not imposed on surgeons. And it reflected not so much surgery's weakness as its strength, because surgery was in a position at that time to pick and choose its own market turf. Although some surgeons embraced the endoscope—especially those in subspecialties accessing their organ systems through a natural orifice, like colon and rectal and ear, nose, and throat (ENT) surgeons—most left it alone, preferring to concentrate their efforts exclusively on those procedures that demanded the craft skills for which they had invested heavily (Surg 1985).

The shift from diagnostic to operative endoscopic applications forced general surgeons to change their orientation. Some surgeons, especially those who, for whatever reason, became attracted to the potential of the endoscope early on, published commentary in the major surgical journals arguing that only surgeons should administer the new operative endoscopic techniques. They pleaded with their colleagues to develop a greater interest in the endoscope's potential (AJS 1976b; ArchS 1973a–e; SGO 1973, 1975). However, rank-and-file surgeons typically ignored such calls until the scope encroached upon their market territory. Then, they challenged the efficacy of its treatment outcomes and attempted to draw strong lines of demarcation between the endoscopic and the surgical procedures to which they were committed (AnnS 1971, 332; CJS 1994a, 273; SCNA 1989a, 1129).

As this response proved inadequate, and as gastroenterologists became more and more aggressive in crossing these demarcation lines, general surgery embraced the endoscope as its own and attempted to legitimate surgeons' right to perform operative endoscopy alongside of the gastroenterologists. The American Board of Surgery, in 1980 in a revision to its residency training guidelines, called upon surgical residency programs to provide their charges with familiarity and performance training in endoscopic procedures. However, the performance clause was removed from these guidelines in 1981, after residency directors complained that they did not have the resources to offer endoscopic training to all residents (SGO 1982, 1990; Surg 1983a, 180; see also ArchS 1990b, 148). The Society of American Gastrointestinal Endoscopic Surgeons (SAGES) was also incorporated in 1981 as an association of surgeons dedicated to establishing and preserving their rights to perform endoscopy (SCNA 1989a, 1989c). In his 1985 presidential address to the Central Surgical Association, Dr. Lloyd Nyhus, defining operative endoscopy as one of four important but neglected areas of general surgery development, called on surgery departments to beef up endoscopic training in their residencies (Surg 1985, 621; SCNA 1989a). As more surgeons heeded these calls, heated, partisan debate broke out over which specialty had the legitimate claim to perform operative gastrointestinal endoscopy.

Gastroenterology's Closure Argument

When general surgeons began to take up fiber-optic endoscopy in greater numbers in the 1980s, gastroenterologists questioned their sudden interest in an instrument that they themselves had developed and controlled almost unilaterally, and without contest, up until that point. One response, emanating mostly from academic medicine, was friendly. Recognizing the symbiotic interdependencies the specialties historically had shared with each other, this response attempted to ease the growing tension with the sharing of endoscopy suites. The leitmotiv of this position was stated succinctly in the following gastroenterological commentary: "No single discipline should attempt to claim proprietorship of gastrointestinal endoscopy. In medicine, there is no place for sibling rivalry" (AJG 1985c, 658; see also SCNA 1989c).

However, endoscopy had blurred traditional lines of demarcation between medicine and surgery. And, because of this, it became very difficult to sustain or revert to the conventions of the past. Endoscopy made it possible to combine diagnosis and surgical treatment in a single time-bound procedure that could not be neatly fragmented. It was very difficult to anticipate, prior to scoping the patient, what course of action—surgical, medical, or endoscopic—would be called for in treating the case. Hence, there was no easy formula for dividing up endoscopy cases between surgeons and gastroenterologists. Doing so would inevitably provoke contention. Once endoscopy began to revolutionize medical practice, there was no turning back to the easier days when turf definitions were widely shared and maintained.

This blurring of the traditional boundary between medicine and surgery led some to propose the creation of an amalgamated superspecialty that combined all facets of gastrointestinal medicine—that is, abdominal surgery, gastrointestinal endoscopy, and internal medicine. This superspecialty would take responsibility for diagnosis and for all treatments for gastrointestinal conditions. Those advocating this radical proposal looked to the hybrid specialties of urology and gynecology as their model (AJS 1983b, 2; ArchS 1994a;

NEJM 1992b, 1627; Surg 1988, 117). Though provocative, and perhaps sensible, such calls were not readily heeded by either specialty. The trust and commitment required to meld institutionally these very different occupational cultures were quite difficult to generate (see AJS 1980e, 7).

The second response taken by gastroenterologists was to argue for strict closure around all gastrointestinal endoscopic procedures. This response was partisan and provoked considerable contention. General surgeons defined it as shamelessly self-interested and unduly repressive, as expressed in the following surgical commentary:

> Flexible fiberoptic gastrointestinal endoscopy became the new mainstay of gastroenterologists, and the practice of gastroenterology changed abruptly. With the changes emerged a new breed of procedure-oriented medical practitioner, whose zeal created a whole new set of problems for surgeon endoscopists. . . . With time, the rank and file of practicing gastroenterologists—whose numbers had grown impressively, perhaps because of the glamour and economic potential of flexible endoscopy—began to manifest turf consciousness. Economic considerations continued to mount, adding to the political swirl, and in an unprecedented manner, attempts were made to restrict surgeon endoscopists' opportunities. . . . The collective spirit of the multidisciplinary pioneers drowned in waves of greed and ego. (SCNA 1989c, 1124; see also AJG 1984a, 909; AJS 1991l, 400–401)

However, there was logic to gastroenterology's response. The supervised training for endoscopy in gastroenterology fellowship programs was quite rigorous. In order to attain technical competence in the procedure, the Federation of Digestive Diseases suggested that each candidate perform a minimum of fifty gastroscopies, fifty colonoscopies, and twenty-five polypectomies under immediate supervision. The American Society of Gastroenterological Endoscopists (ASGE) suggested even more: one hundred gastroscopies, one hundred colonoscopies, and twenty polypectomies (AIM 1993a, 1993b; AJS 1980e, 1982; for requirements in Britain, see GUT 1987). Although recognizing the variable nature of skill acquisition and case opportunities in residencies and, therefore, refusing to mandate specific numbers, the American Board of Internal Medicine established guidelines in 1977 for training gastroenterology fellows in its two-year fellowship programs. These guidelines specified that such programs provide training in diagnostic and therapeutic endoscopy, including upper gastrointestinal endoscopy and biopsy; colonoscopy, biopsy, and polypectomy; dilation procedures for esophageal disease; small intestinal biopsy; and percutaneous liver biopsy. These guidelines also called for familiarity, but not necessarily technical proficiency, in the more advanced endoscopic techniques, including the operative procedures associated with ERCP and laparoscopy. Later, the American Board of Internal Medicine and the Board of Gastroenterology extended its evaluation of clinical endoscopic skills beyond written examinations. It began to ask fellowship directors to evaluate directly in writing the specific procedural skills of their charges (AJG 1987c; see also AJG 1984e, 322). Gastroenterologists, having invested heavily in learning these techniques, were outraged when other physicians and surgeons began to apply for endoscopic privileges in their hospitals without undergoing comparable training.

In 1984, Dr. James L. Achord, an academic gastroenterologist, published an incendiary editorial in the *American Journal of Gastroenterology*, titled "Who Said Surgeons Had to be Trained in Gastrointestinal Endoscopy?" (AJG 1984e). Gastroenterologists had traditionally advised hospital committees to grant endoscopic privileges to specialists who either learned endoscopy in rigorous residency or fellowship programs in gastroenterology, colon and rectal surgery, or general surgery, or who had equivalent experience. At that time, the primary concern was to exclude general practitioners or nursing assistants from moving into endoscopic markets (see, for example, JAMA 1981b). Surgeons, often dependent on gastroenterologists for referrals, were not so threatening early on, especially because so few of them showed any interest in gastrointestinal endoscopy during its development as a diagnostic instrument.

This benign response to the surgeon-endoscopists changed as the latter began to embrace the scope for operative applications. Achord's commentary spelled out a strong argument for why only those trained in gastroenterology should do gastrointestinal endoscopy, an argument that set off a round of polemics regarding the credentialing of endoscopic privileges in hospitals. Achord expressed alarm that surgeons, and others, were attempting to perform endoscopy without the level of supervised training demanded in gastroenterology's fellowship programs. He called for the application of the rigorous standards set by the ASGE to all those seeking hospital privileges in gastrointestinal endoscopy (AJG 1984e, 322; 1985a). Although the

American Board of Surgery called for familiarity with endoscopy in its revised training guidelines, this was not enough to insure that general surgeons had become competent endoscopists (AJG 1984e, 1985a; see also AJG 1984a). As surgeon commentators attested, Achord's proposal would essentially force all surgeons, before they could become credentialed as endoscopists, to enroll in gastroenterological fellowship programs.

In calling for the extension of gastroenterology's strict training standards to all endoscopists, Achord argued that, although the technical requirements for simply passing the scope could be learned rather quickly for many procedures, acquiring the skill needed for adequately interpreting, diagnosing, and treating anatomy required long training and experience. He further argued that surgeons' craft skills did not translate easily into the skills required to perform diagnostic and therapeutic endoscopy. After all, endoscopy accesses the abdominal cavity from within the organ system, while surgeons do so externally through the open abdominal cavity. Surgeons rarely see the inside of the organs they treat until these are dissected or resected. Achord scoffed at the argument that surgeons' limited experiences in these latter functions adequately prepared them for doing endoscopy.

Achord also questioned surgeons' motives. He claimed that 90 percent of endoscopy did not involve a surgical consideration. In making claims for unilaterally controlling the scope, Achord pointed out that gastroenterologists, as diagnosticians, routinely managed patients with a range of gastrointestinal illnesses. He also noted that gastroenterologists were quick to refer their patients to surgeons when surgical treatment was called for on the endoscopic examination. In response to calls for interspecialty endoscopy suites, Achord claimed that the specialties of medicine and surgery bred contradictory personalities and that these personalities could not be expected to share endoscopy suites without conflict (AJG 1984e, 323). In short, Achord argued that there was no need for surgeons to take up endoscopy.

Achord's editorials defended the recent line of demarcation that had developed between gastroenterology and surgery. If heeded, his proposals would have secured gastroenterologists' de facto monopoly over the diagnostic and therapeutic endoscopic techniques that they pioneered.

General Surgery's Response

To legitimate their embrace of the scope, general surgeons countered this logic. Addressing the medical profession generally, and hospital committees granting access privileges in particular, surgeons argued that gastroenterologists had exaggerated the difficulty of endoscopic techniques and that surgeons' special training and hands-on experiences in the open abdomen enabled them quite easily to pick up the new skills required in passing the scope and in interpreting anatomy through it. Surgeons argued, moreover, that their training and experiences better qualified them for operative endoscopy than their internist counterparts.

First, surgeons argued that endoscopy was not a new procedure for the surgical specialties. Some hybrid surgical specialties, like urology, and some surgical subspecialties, like thoracic, colon and rectal, and ENT surgery, pioneered the use of the earlier rigid endoscopes many decades before the advent of fiber-optic endoscopy. Internists and gastroenterologists, prior to fiber optics, would often refer patients to these surgical specialists if an endoscopic procedure was indicated. A few innovative general surgeons also worked alongside the gastroenterologists at the cutting edge of the fiber-optic technology, developing endoscopic applications for surgical conditions, such as the intraoperative approach to locating and removing bile duct stones discussed above. In their commentaries during the 1980s, general surgeons pointed to this earlier period in the development of fiber-optic endoscopy when gastroenterologists and general surgeons had worked together in alleged harmony advancing the technology (AJG 1985b; CurS 1978, 223; SCNA 1989c, 1124). Although not without challenge (AJG 1985a), general surgeons used stories of these historical precedents to legitimate their endoscopy program during the 1980s.

Surgeons also argued that the interpretive skills needed for localizing anatomy and interpreting its condition were similar in the open surgical and endoscopic modalities. Their hands-on experiences treating tissue, coupled with the direct panoramic view provided in their treatment modality, gave surgeons an advantage in mastering the intricacies of endoscopy that other physicians lacked. Because of this, surgeons argued that they did not require the same number of trials to hone their proficiency in this technique as did those coming

to endoscopy from specialties lacking direct access to the organ systems they treated. As stated in the following surgical commentary:

> The surgeon, in the course of 5 or more years of residency training, reg-
> ularly holds, cuts into, exposes, and inspects the interior; resects;
> replaces; and repairs the hollow smooth-muscle viscera of the gas-
> trointestinal tract. The resulting familiarity with the anatomy, tex-
> ture, resilience, compliance, and strength of tissues, as well as with
> gross lesions, is an enormous advantage and confers an advanced
> standing on the surgeon as a student endoscopist. The surgeon's po-
> tential for learning endoscopy is clearly superior, and the number of
> endoscopic procedures carried out thus is not crucial. (SCNA 1989c,
> 1125)

Finally, surgeons argued that they were in the best position to interpret the findings of the endoscopic examination prior to surgical
treatment. One concern expressed in surgical commentary was that
the information provided to the operating surgeon in the endoscopy
reports prepared by gastroenterologists was often insufficiently detailed for surgical purposes. This was spelled out in the following surgical commentary:

> [The gastroenterologist] has never found himself in the awkward po-
> sition of the surgeon who requires precise knowledge of the exact dis-
> tance of the rectal lesion from the anal verge or the position of the
> cardioesophageal junction, and who discovers that these or other im-
> portant anatomical descriptions are lacking from an endoscopist's re-
> port. (AJG 1985b, 232)

The root of this problem was that gastroenterologists, from the
point of view of general surgeons, lacked the detailed, nuanced
knowledge of anatomy required to assist in an optimal manner. To
rectify this, one surgical commentator argued that if gastroenterologists were not willing to spend one or two years in surgical training
to acquire the requisite operative knowledge, then surgeons should
perform their own endoscopies (see AJG 1985b).

Surgeons argued that their particular training and orientation better prepared them to assess the case and to make the treatment decision. After all, surgeons were trained to make quick assessments
on the spot. Gastroenterologists, on the other hand, were trained to
consult first, and typically did so when surgical conditions were in-

dicated (AJG 1984a, 907). Surgeons argued that operative cases could be treated more effectively if they themselves performed endoscopy and made the necessary decisions on the spot, hence removing the intermediary bottleneck—the gastroenterologist—from the decision-making process altogether.

Surgeons argued, moreover, that they were better equipped to deal with the complications associated with operative endoscopy. Although rare, complications such as perforation and hemorrhaging could call for emergency treatment and have life-threatening consequences. Gastroenterologists, with no training in traditional surgical procedures, could not respond immediately to such complications. Their only option is to recognize such complications quickly and call immediately for the surgeon to treat them in an emergency setting. General surgeons, on the other hand, are trained to treat such conditions. They are better able to recognize conditions that cause such complications, to avoid them, and to react to them in a timely fashion when they occur. Surgeons argued that having surgeons, rather than internists, performing operative endoscopy would reduce the incidence of these complications, as well as their morbidity and mortality rates (AJG 1984a, 907).

Structural Impediments

Structural impediments, however, confronted general surgeons when they attempted to embrace the gastrointestinal endoscope during the 1980s. The results of a survey of the chairs of general surgery departments published in 1982 reported that only 30 percent offered a formal endoscopy program in their residency training, and only 29 percent offered informal training. Only about half of those offering either type of training reported that all of their residents received it. Fourteen percent reported that gastroenterology monopolized the endoscopy service at their institutions. Half thought that the gastroenterology service could not meet the training demands of general surgery (AJS 1982). Surgical commentary increasingly criticized the quality of endoscopic training offered to general surgery residents in gastroenterology services. They increasingly called for dedicated surgical endoscopy suites, supervised by surgeon endoscopists, to meet the specific training needs of surgical residents (AJS 1982; AmS 1989a; AnnS 1986b; SCNA 1989a).

General surgeons' attempt to drive a wedge into the endoscopic market proved an uphill struggle. Their successes were limited ones at best. As late as 1989, one commentary reported that only 15 percent of general surgery residencies had established formal surgical endoscopy training, and much of the training received was still heavily influenced and controlled by gastroenterologists (SCNA 1989a, 1129). The Society of American Gastrointestinal Endoscopic Surgeons grew during the 1980s and had over one thousand members in 1989. However, this constituted only a fraction of the over 30,000 general surgeons in practice and in residency. Gastroenterology's counterpart organization—ASGE—was three to four times larger and held a much more influential position in the specialty.

Most importantly, gastroenterology's upstream position in medicine's intraoccupational division of labor helped it to secure its control over its endoscopic markets. General surgery could not break gastroenterology's grip over these markets from its disadvantaged downstream position in the division of labor. Once gastroenterologists had established themselves in the 1970s as the rightful heirs to the gastrointestinal endoscope, and once surgeons ceded them this right by their own neglect of the fiber-optic scope's development and application, arguments and rhetoric, no matter what their logic, proved to be rather impotent weapons in reasserting dominance over surgical turf. Gastroenterologists had long been recognized throughout the profession as the more accomplished endoscopists, and gastroenterologists saw the bulk of the referrals sent out for endoscopy from fellow internists and general practitioners.[2]

For all the pronouncements and rhetoric emanating from general surgery's leaders, the timing of general surgery's foray into surgical endoscopy proved unfortunate. General surgeons were simply not in a strong structural position for dislodging an opponent from a burgeoning market, a market that surgeons had initially chosen to neglect and even abandon. By the time they realized their strategic mistake, it was much too late for them to secure access to this market. And, by the 1980s, general surgeons no longer had the moral authority within the occupation to influence the decisions made there by others. General surgeons could do little more than watch their markets shrink, as gastroenterology extended the reach of its endoscopes to accommodate the market interests of its growing legions.[3] In the late 1980s general surgery's position within the medical profession's intraoccupational division of labor was probably weaker than at any point in the twentieth century. Its future prospects appeared dim (JAMA 1989a).

Notes

1. The argument that operative workloads were not high enough to hone and maintain superior surgical skills is related to this as well. This concern has been addressed since the 1970s (see NEJM 1973a, 1973b, 1976a, 1981d).

2. Recognizing this, some argued in surgical commentary (SCNA 1989c, 1125) that surgeon endoscopists should increase their visibility to students in the earlier years of their medical school training.

3. In the 1990s, gastroenterologists shifted their focus from their boundary with general surgery to their boundary with a potentially more formidable threat working upstream in medicine's intraoccupational division of labor—general and family practitioners. The American Academy of Family Physicians allegedly offered short courses in endoscopy for family physicians during its 1992 meeting. Fearing that this development might shift endoscopy suites from the hospitals, where gastroenterologists had considerable influence, to the general practitioners' private offices, the AGA, the ASGE, and the ACG all issued position statements that advocated limiting reimbursement to only those who had attained hospital credentials to perform endoscopy. The ACG also circulated a memorandum to hospitals on the legal risks of credentialing inadequately trained physicians. Gastroenterologists called for restricting scope privileges to those who were board certified in gastroenterology, or who were board certified in other specialties with "commensurate knowledge, training, and experience in gastrointestinal endoscopy." The governing societies of gastroenterology acted very vigorously to nip this challenge in the bud. They argued, once again, that although the technical requirements for completing some endoscopic procedures could be mastered in a relatively short time, the cognitive and interpretive components could not be so easily acquired (see AJG 1993e; Gas 1993a).

8

Technological Innovation
in the Surgical Craft

The first wave of innovative operative procedures in gastroenterological endoscopy, and also in interventional radiology, wedged their way into surgical markets by taking over procedures that can best be defined as peripheral. General surgeons' core procedures were, by and large, left untouched by these early developments. Before the 1980s, for example, few were willing to question—let alone challenge—surgeons' control over the treatment of gallbladder diseases. After all, surgeons had delivered stellar results here for over one hundred years. Surgeons often used their success in treating gallbladder diseases as the reference case in talking up their occupational virtues. One radiologist claimed in gastroenterological commentary that, as an arena for innovation and experimentation, gallbladder diseases were "virtually 'off-limits'" because of surgeons' dominance over this segment of the anatomy (GCNA 1991b, 209).

However, by the late 1980s, "off-limits" was no longer acceptable as a defense of time-honored surgical turf. And internists began developing new threats to general surgery's hold on the treatment of gallbladder disease. Although still in experimental stages, nonsurgical treatments, such as bile-acid therapy, contact dissolution techniques, and percutaneous approaches to stone removal, were expanding. Extracorporeal shock-wave lithotripsy was also being developed to break up gallstones in the biliary tract without surgery (ArchS 1989b; Gas 1989a; GCNA 1991a, 1991c). Surgeons responded to this development with deep concern, as expressed in the following surgical commentary:

> Surgeons have been receiving the news of lithotripsy for gallstones with anxiety and some disdain. The initial pieces of the story have seemed to be a rewrite of the advent of endoscopy, biliary stinting for pancreatic cancer, endoscopic polypectomy, and percutaneous drainage of abdominal abscesses. The possibility that an operation done by surgeons since 1882 may be replaced by a procedure not involving an incision, and that this procedure may not be done by surgeons, is disconcerting to say the least. . . . As distasteful as it may be to some, we must now acknowledge that the procedure from which our patients may benefit in the future may not always involve an incision, sponges, scissors, or sutures. (ArchS 1989b, 769–70; see also CJS 1990)

For a time, it looked as if gallbladder removal, one of surgery's bread-and-butter procedures for over one hundred years, might suffer the same fate as open surgeries lost to other nonsurgical specialties. Losing gallbladder diseases probably would have dealt a knockout blow to general surgery's already deflated prestige, as well as to the livelihoods of many of its practitioners. The threat of nonsurgical approaches to this procedure, both materially and symbolically, shook general surgery's raison d'être. This time, however, general surgeons countered these foreboding threats with a bold technological innovation of their own.

Laparoscopic Innovation for Gallbladder Removal

The first successful laparoscopic gallbladder removal is generally credited to a French surgeon with extensive experience in gynecological laparoscopy, who performed the technique in 1987 and who did not publicize his results. The procedure was picked up and refined one year later by surgeons in Bordeaux. These surgeons promoted the procedure's use worldwide (see, for example, AJS 1993f, 444; ArchS 1990a; SCNA 1994d).[1]

An American variant of the laparoscopic gallbladder approach was performed in 1988. The American pioneers worked in teams consisting of a surgeon and a gynecologist: Eddie Joe Reddick and James Daniell in Nashville; Barry McKernan and William Saye in Atlanta

(AJS 1991m; for technical differences between approaches, see AJS 1993f). Reddick and a second partner, Douglas Olsen, are credited generally with popularizing the American technique (SCNA 1992, 655). Nashville and Atlanta quickly became centers of laser laparoscopic developments. As the word spread, American general surgeons quickly embraced the innovation and flocked to short courses to learn it.

Politically, the timing of this innovation could not have been better. After considerable turf losses for over two decades, and in the face of challenges to one of their bread-and-butter procedures, general surgeons could for the first time offer a "minimally invasive" procedure of their own to patients. This procedure could better compete with the alternatives to open surgery on patient friendly terms—less scarring, minimal hospitalization, less post-operative pain, quicker recoveries, and the like (AJS 1990b, 1991e, 1991i; SCNA 1994e). Once this new, patient-friendly technology entered local surgical markets, surgeons felt compelled to learn it in order to sustain their viability there (see ArchS 1990a, 1245). Even the pioneering surgeons recognized that the motivation for adopting this technique was primarily economic, as stated in the following surgical commentary:

> For years, non-surgeons have been eroding the practice of general surgery. This has never been more evident than with the invasion of lithotripsy and dissolution therapy on gallbladder disease. The emergence of laparoscopic laser cholecystectomy has given surgeons a chance to reclaim their territory with a relatively noninvasive operation, and surgeons are flocking to the procedure in droves. (AJS 1990a, 488)

Thus, open gallbladder removal, a procedure that had been performed with laudable results for over a century, was displaced as the procedure of choice for gallbladder disease rather quickly by a new laparoscopic application developed by general surgeons themselves. Once they took the plunge, general surgeons began to boast of their newfound capacity for innovation, a capacity that they used judiciously in shoring up their market position. Laparoscopic gallbladder surgery, more than any other development in the 1990s, helped to salvage general surgery's market position and reputation, as expressed in the following surgical commentary:

The "abdominable surgeons" live on! Laparoscopic cholecystectomy, a consumer-driven procedure, has engulfed our profession and challenged our creativity while increasing the visibility and viability of general surgery. . . . Many predict this to be a delightful beginning. For the senior (mature) members of our profession, this may sound like "Star Wars," but it has the aura of permanency. A decade of poor professional recognition and diminished pride in general surgery has been reversed. (ArchS 1991a, 1335)

In developing an occupational program for the new approach, general surgery, by and large, learned from its belated attempt to incorporate gastrointestinal endoscopy into its domain. Not only did general surgeons take de facto control over the laparoscope early on, they drew upon their own time-honored legitimation principles in establishing effective closure over the technique's extension into their markets.

Strain, Struggle, and Uncertainty

In the United States, medical-research complexes and community hospitals developed to fulfill different functional needs. The medical-research complexes developed with a mandate to engage in research and improve health care. In these institutions accomplishments in research and in developing innovative approaches earned the status and monetary rewards faculty coveted. The community hospitals, on the other hand, served the immediate health care needs of the community. Practical successes in the provision of services earned the monetary and status rewards valued by private practitioners. Typically, new innovations were developed in the medical-research complexes, subjected to clinical trials and publication reviews, and from there diffused out to the community hospitals (AJS 1993g, 536).

This course was reversed in the case of laparoscopic gallbladder removal. General surgery, by and large, did not take an interest in laparoscopy's prevideo developments. And the initial reception for laparoscopic gallbladder removal from academic surgery was lukewarm at best, as evidenced in the following surgical commentary from one of the technology's French pioneers: "Laparoscopic cholecystectomy had a semiclandestine debut in nonacademic settings with the initial reviews being highly critical, incredulous, and strongly sarcastic" (AJS 1991h, 408; 1993f, 444).

Some academic surgeons, leery of the hype surrounding the new technology and questioning its rightful place in general surgery, attempted to expropriate surgical laparoscopy's early development from its community hospital base. They planned to subject the new procedure to controlled clinical trials, arguing that until the new technology proved itself in controlled experimental settings, it should not be offered as a procedure of choice in the community hospitals (see, for example, AJS 1990d). Some argued that before the laparoscopic procedure could be considered as a viable alternative, its mortality and morbidity rates must equal or better those achieved with the standard surgical approach (AJS 1993h; see also AJS 1991o, 401–402). Had they been implemented, such strict standards could well have choked off the development and diffusion of the laparoscopic approach, given that the morbidity and mortality rates of the open-incision procedure had undergone considerable refinement over its one-hundred-plus year history (ArchS 1992c; see also AJS 1989a; SCNA 1994d). However, with rapid diffusion of the new technology taking place largely outside of their institutional base, academic surgeons increasingly realized that they lacked the power to accomplish their designs. They could not influence the community practitioners or slow the new technology's spread (AJS 1991o, 401–402).

Early Promise of Surgical Laparoscopy

The surgical laparoscopists' early successes with gallbladder removal emboldened them. Like the gastroenterological endoscopists before them, they quickly began to push the envelope with the new technology. In skilled hands, the laparoscope could accomplish many of the same outcomes as open-incision techniques. Unlike with open surgery, however, laparoscopy could compete with other minimally invasive procedures on patient-friendly terms (AJS 1990e). Laparoscopic surgeons reported their successes with much enthusiasm and aplomb.

Early studies claimed documented treatment outcomes with the laparoscopic approach that were comparable to those produced with open surgery (AJS 1992b; AnnS 1991). Initially, laparoscopic surgeons avoided difficult cases, because the limitations of the laparoscopic modality made it difficult to identify structures and to manage tissue from a distance (see chapter 1). Cases with sepsis, acute organ or tissue inflammation, common bile duct stones, prior upper abdominal operations, or a major bleeding source were not treated laparoscopically (AJS 1991n). However, as their skills improved, some surgeons began to tackle these more difficult cases through the laparoscope as well. Cases with acute inflammation, for example, were performed laparoscopically by some highly skilled surgeons with a reported success rate that was comparable to open surgeries. Laparoscopic surgeons argued, in the face of criticism, that acute inflammation in skilled hands was not a counterindication for the technique (AJG 1993c; AJS 1991a, 1991m; for criticisms, see AJG 1993d).

Enterprising laparoscopists quickly began to explore the use of the laparoscopic approach to regain turf lost to gastroenterology. One of the most important of these was the management of stones lodged in the biliary ducts. One report claimed that 90 percent of the stones found in the common bile duct could be removed laparoscopically during gallbladder surgery through the cystic duct, reducing much of the need for gastroenterologists to perform pre- or postoperative ERCP (AJS 1993e). Surgeons also reported using the laparoscopic approach in stomach surgeries, such as managing malignant duodenal obstructions and peptic ulcerations (AJS 1991k; BJS 1993c, 1994). In short order, laparoscopy promised to halt the postwar erosion of these surgical markets.

Enterprising surgeons also began to explore the use of the laparoscopic approach in performing other bread-and-butter procedures—that is, appendectomy and hernia repair (see BJS 1992, 1993a; DCR 1993b). The laparoscopic approach was used further in small bowel resection; colon resections; and the removal of spleens, adrenal glands, kidneys, uteruses, and lymph glands; and lung resections, among other procedures (see AJS 1993g). Although the laparoscopic proponents defined such extensions as natural, they threatened to disrupt established surgical markets by shifting patient demand away from the established surgical guard. Surgeons responded critically to these reports (BJS 1993b, 1993c), arguing for restricting these extensions of the technology to academic institutions and submitting their results to controlled clinical trials (ArchS 1991b, 1992b).

Even with all of the reported successes, surgical commentators expressed a good deal of unease about the rapid spread of the laparoscopic techniques. Even laparoscopy's surgical proponents expressed concern over the laparoscopic approach's rapid diffusion. These pioneers, through their own experiences, realized that special skills were required for performing surgery through the scope and that the learning curve involved in acquiring these skills could not be mastered on the cheap (see chapters 1 and 2). They realized that the laparoscope and the laser were dangerous in the hands of inexperienced and untrained surgeons and that catastrophic consequences would not bode well for the future of the technique. As Reddick stated in surgical commentary:

> In our hurry to jump on the bandwagon, we must ensure that each surgeon who performs this operation is adequately trained. This operation is very instrument-dependent and requires not only a knowledge of the instrumentation, but also a relearning of hand-eye coordination. If poorly trained scope surgeons cause a high percentage of complications, this excellent addition to our surgical offerings will quickly get a bad reputation and could be highly restricted. (AJS 1990a, 488; see also AJS 1990d, 1991o)

A major concern was the high level of skill required. The surgeons who were pushing the laparoscopic envelope, and reporting their impressive successes in the surgical journals, were all virtuoso performers. They could do marvelous work. However, some questioned the extent to which the average surgeon, brand-new to the technique, could be expected to achieve the same success. To the skeptics, the critical question was not what was possible but what was reasonable to expect from the legions of surgeons newly embracing the scope in response to market pressures (AJS 1990b, 489). What would the results be if rank-and-file surgeons began to overextend themselves, attempting complicated procedures beyond the range of their training and existing skill levels? This question was soon answered—not in rhetoric—but in outcomes documented by the New York State Health Department.

Delegitimation Threat

The initial reports of serious complications came from surgeons who had repaired bile duct injuries of some of the early laparoscopic patients. These injuries were often quite severe. Surgeons in San

Diego early on reported reconstructing the biliary tracts of six laparoscopic patients. They were struck by the damage caused by the indiscriminate use of the laser in this region. Tissue was vaporized to the point where reconstruction was quite difficult. These surgeons also noted cases of injury to vascular structures as well. Shocked by these results, these surgeons also called for the restriction of the technique to the university centers until clinical trials could test its viability. They attributed most of the damage done to younger inexperienced surgeons (ArchS 1991c). Surgeons from the Lahey Clinic in Boston also reported receiving over twenty cases of bile duct injuries after the introduction of the technique. Such injuries were very rare in the open procedure. Later surgical commentary would typically mention this initial rash of bile duct injuries, discuss how to avoid them, and claim that the situation had improved as surgeons' learning curves progressed (SCNA 1994b). The threat of these catastrophes to the fate of this technology, however, was very real. As Renée Fox and Judith Swazey (1978, chap. 5) have pointed out, moratoriums on the use of promising therapeutic innovations have occurred repeatedly in the history of medicine and surgery.

Unfortunately, such mishaps are quite common with new procedures. However, the situation in the first few years of the laparoscopic gallbladder approach appears to have been exceptionally trying. Three developments contributed to this. First, the NYS Health Department, because of a statewide planning and research system established in 1979, kept empirical documentation on the outcomes of the new technique. The NYS Health Department began to look closely at the results of this particular procedure after being alerted to its potential pitfalls by the editor of the *American Journal of Surgery*. The editor became gravely concerned over the horror stories circulating about the new technique's complications.

Second, alarmed over the catastrophes it had documented, the NYS Health Department took decisive action to better monitor and regulate the credentialing process in New York state. The Health Department sent a memorandum to all hospitals in the state spelling out minimal training requirements for the new technique. These requirements included, after an introduction to the basics of the technique, a minimum of fifteen procedures conducted under the supervision of a certified laparoscopic surgeon. This move was unprecedented. States typically had granted hospitals, and the medical professionals running them, unilateral authority to establish their own criteria for granting operating privileges. The conclusion reached by the NYS Health Department, after reviewing the data, was that the traditional safeguards were no longer adequate for protecting patients from the potential hazards of new surgical technologies.

Third, after lauding the benefits of the new "key-hole" surgery, the press reported these mishaps to the public in what some surgeons viewed as a sensationalistic fashion. These reports generated a scandal for the new technology, holding it to a critical level of public and media scrutiny that was rare for a medical innovation (see ATU 1992a–e; NYT 1992).

In a 1993 report published in the *American Journal of Surgery* representatives from the NYS Health Department explained their actions to the surgical community (AJS 1993b). They reported the statistical irregularities that had forced their hand. They first noted a suspicious increase in the number of gallbladder removals performed since the advent of the laparoscopic approach, increases that probably had more to do with competitive forces than with medical ones. Even more alarming were the reports of serious complications. From August 1990 to March 1992, 158 serious incidents involving laparoscopic gallbladder surgeries occurred in 85 of the 268 hospitals operating in New York state. This number probably underreported the true incident rate, because many hospitals failed to report the information requested. Of these complications 34 percent involved the leakage of bile in the abdomen; 22 percent involved damage to the bile duct; and 19 percent involved hemorrhage. Oftentimes, these complications lay hidden in the closed abdomen and were not found until days after the surgery was completed. Several patients died, and their deaths triggered legal actions (AJS 1993b; see also ATU 1992c; Lancet 1993b).

The new credentialing guidelines had a twofold purpose. First and foremost they were to protect the innocent public from the hands of inexperienced and naive operators, who themselves were being unduly influenced by market pressures and the hype of the instrument manufacturers. Second, they were intended to save from disrepute a promising new procedure. Had the initial mishaps continued, authorities might have decided to close down the laparoscopic procedure completely. To salvage the new technique, the NYS Health Department felt forced to regulate its use. Later reports acknowledged the failure of general surgery's regulatory bodies to introduce and monitor the new laparoscopic technique in an effective fashion during its infancy (ArchS 1992a, 403).

Establishing Monopoly Closure

During the initial wave of enthusiasm over the new procedure it appeared that general surgeons had learned from their trying experience with gastrointestinal endoscopy. Rather than stand on the sidelines while a competitor developed turf-threatening technology, general surgeons were at the forefront of this development. Rank-and-file general surgeons flocked to the laparoscopic technique early on in unprecedented fashion. According to the NYS Health Department, two-thirds of all gallbladders removed in the state of New York were done laparoscopically by 1992. Emboldened by their advances in extending the range of video laparoscopy's applications, general surgeons boasted of their newfound capacity for innovation. This technology's impressive introduction enabled them to face their future with hope rather than despair.

However, the rash of well-publicized early mishaps threatened all that this new technology had promised. Had general surgery failed to develop an effective program for monitoring the training and credentialing of surgeons in this new approach, it could well have lost its control over the laparoscope. Gynecologists potentially stood as a competitor to general surgeons' control over this instrument and its surgical applications. After all, gynecologists pioneered the development of prevideo laparoscopy; the medical community had long recognized gynecologists as those with advanced laparoscopic skills; and the refined skills of gynecologists were essential to the initial stages of the gallbladder innovation. Indeed, some gynecologists reportedly had applied early on for hospital privileges to remove gallbladders laparoscopically (AJS 1991o, 401). Given their bitter turf losses at the hands of those promoting other new technologies, general surgeons watched this development with considerable alarm.

Gastroenterologists could also have stood as potential competitors to general surgeons' control over the laparoscope. Gastroenterology, never bashful in embracing new technology, had also developed some interest in laparoscopy early on for diagnosis and for liver biopsy. The Board of Gastroenterology, prior to the advent of laparoscopic gallbladder surgery, had listed laparoscopy as one of the procedures in which its residents should be trained. Whatever its objective basis, the threat of encroachment from such formidable competitors was thought to be real in the surgical community. It motivated general surgeons to act aggressively and proactively in defense of time-honored turf.

Training and Credentialing Standards

General surgery developed an occupational program to counter these potentially turf-threatening developments. At the most basic level, this program established requirements for the training and credentialing of general surgeons in laparoscopic procedures. SAGES was one of the first surgical bodies to offer training standards. SAGES discouraged hospital committees from granting laparoscopic privileges to surgeons taking only one of the instrument manufacturer's short courses. SAGES recommended that general surgeons first observe diagnostic laparoscopies in order to learn the basic steps of the procedure, then perform at least ten procedures under the direct supervision of a certified laparoscopic surgeon, and then complete a formal course, preferably from an accredited residency. Such a rigorous training and credentialing program was thought necessary for establishing the legitimacy of both the laparoscopic gallbladder procedure itself and general surgeons' control over it. As Reddick stated in reference to the SAGES guidelines, "Although this may seem a bit intense for a board-certified surgeon, it is imperative that we avoid sabotaging our success at getting the gallbladder back into our specialty by allowing poorly trained surgeons to create a broad base of complications that might ultimately destroy laparoscopic laser cholecystectomy" (AJS 1990a, 488; see also AJS 1991f).

In response to the initial rash of mishaps, hospital credentialing committees did become more diligent, and surgeons' laparoscopic skills did improve. Residencies also began to offer more effective training in laparoscopic approaches, responding in innovative ways to the peculiar skill demands of the technique (see AJS 1992a; SCNA 1994c; SGO 1992). General surgery, because of its efforts to correct the initial wave of mishaps with the new technology, neither discredited laparoscopic gallbladder removal nor lost its grip on the video laparoscope. In the fall of 1992, shortly after the initial wave of negative media reports, a panel from the National Institutes of

Health endorsed laparoscopic gallbladder removal as the procedure of choice for treating gallbladder diseases (ATU 1992a).

General surgery's occupational program did more than simply provide improved training and credentialing standards, however. This program extended general surgery's monopoly claim over laparoscopic gallbladder removal to all of the operative laparoscopic procedures that its practitioners traditionally performed in the open-incision modality. This occupational program legitimated surgeons' control over the laparoscope with a peculiar form of the reduction strategy that Andrew Abbott discusses in *The System of Professions* (1988). This reduction strategy coupled the rhetoric of cognitive abstraction with surgery's time-honored particularistic indeterminacy claim.

Cognitive Abstraction of Craft Skill

Long before the advent of surgical laparoscopy, the definition of surgical virtue had shifted from an emphasis on technique and the development of "good hands" to an emphasis on surgery's more cognitive bases. "Surgical judgment" in interpreting anatomy and in planning appropriate procedures became lauded as the ultimate core virtue of the clinical surgeon. Procedural skills, although essential to effective surgery, were typically downplayed as routinizable or defined as mere complements to good cognitive judgment. As William Nolen (1970, 249) said in a popular autobiographical account of his surgical training during the 1960s:

> Removing a stomach, a gall bladder or an appendix can be a difficult job. . . . Still, a reasonably intelligent, moderately adept individual might learn to do any of these jobs in a few months. If you can cut, sew and tie knots, you can operate. When you get down to fundamentals, that's really all there is to the mechanical phase of surgery.
>
> Then what is there about surgery that makes it necessary for a doctor to study for five years? The answer, in a word, is "judgment."
>
> It acquires a long time and a lot of hard work for a doctor to acquire sound surgical judgment. Every time he sees a patient he has to be able to assess and evaluate the history of the patient's illness, the findings on physical examination, the chemical studies of the blood, the results of x-rays and a multitude of other factors; and after weighing all these factors, he has to decide whether to operate or not, what procedure to

use, whether to do the operation immediately or later. And he has to
be right.

Such a definitional shift can be interpreted as a response to the status deflation that general surgery experienced in the postwar period.
Surgery's gatekeepers felt compelled to emphasize the abstract, cognitive bases of surgery's craft foundations so as to compete more effectively in the new research-oriented environment. Although a
long-standing division has existed between so-called "thinking" and
"cutting" doctors (AnnS 1969, 644), the latter label proved especially
disadvantageous to surgeons in the postwar period. It proved disadvantageous in the allocation of medical school resources, in the de-
termination of undergraduate curricula (AnnS 1969, 649; see also
AnnS 1968, 615), and even in the procurement of Medicare re-
imbursements (AJS 1989b). Increasingly on the defensive, general
surgery was forced to restate its cognitive and rhetorical claims to
market turf.

What was the essence of general surgery's cognitive foundation?
How did general surgery defend the legitimacy of its turf claim? According to statements published by the American Board of Surgery
in the 1980s and 1990s, general surgery's theoretical foundation contains the core knowledge needed to treat conditions requiring
anatomical intervention. This core embraces "anatomy, physiology,
metabolism, immunology, nutrition, pathology, wound healing,
shock and resuscitation, intensive care and neoplasia" (AJS 1983a;
1991d, 196; ArchS 1987). This core knowledge base enables the surgeon to claim responsibility for the "diagnosis, preoperative, operative, and postoperative management" of a specific anatomical region
(AJS 1991d, 196). Because of its reliance on this core abstracted
knowledge base, general surgery makes the same claim to being a scientific specialty as its internist competitors (AnnS 1963b, 775).

Yet surgery's treatment modality gives it a unique claim that dif-
ferentiates it from others. Surgery applies scientific knowledge to a
context-dependent case (AnnS 1963b). As discussed in chapter 1, the
raw case material upon which surgeons work is highly variable. Each
patient's anatomy is to some extent unique. There is considerable
variation as to size, shape, texture, and location of basic structures
(see Pinch, Collins, and Carbone 1997). This makes their location,
effects, and relationships to normal structures quite difficult to interpret. Moreover, surgery's treatment modality, unlike most in in-

ternal medicine, involves a very precise procedure (AnnS 1971). Because of this, successful surgery requires accurate on-the-spot, case-based interpretation and judgment (AJS 1988d, 632). To be successful, surgeons' working knowledge of the tissue regions they treat must be extraordinarily detailed and sensitive to complex idiosyncrasies (AnnS 1963a; 1967, 308).

Thus, the nuanced, case-based nature of surgery's knowledge base separates surgeons from other physicians and demands skills that cannot be reduced to generalized treatment regimens or mechanistic diagnostic formulas (AJS 1971b). Although surgery has always employed and demanded this type of knowledge base, its conscious and explicit articulation during the postwar period has generalized it to a more abstract level. This development was not necessary prior to World War II, when clinical surgery's prestige was clearly on the rise and when surgeons held a dominant position in the medical profession's internal division of labor. Abstracting and generalizing surgeons' knowledge base in this fashion could enable them to extend their turf claims to new procedures—like video laparoscopy—that could be shown to demand similar theoretical and cognitive bases. This abstraction, and extension by reduction, was used successfully by surgeons in the 1990s to secure their hold on what remained of their time-honored market turf (for the significance of cognitive abstraction, see Abbott 1988).

Indeterminacy Claim

Unlike the case of other operative technologies, video laparoscopy's diffusion respected the existing division of labor among the established medical and surgical specialties. This outcome was not preordained or determined solely by technical necessity. Alternative scenarios were quite possible and, according to some of the surgical commentary of the period, quite feared. Video laparoscopy, for example, could have given rise to a general, technologically based specialty. However, whatever their merits, such alternatives never materialized. Video laparoscopy, although performed similarly from operation to operation, was embraced by each of the established surgical specialties for those specific operations to which they already had laid claim. Gynecologists used it for treatment of the uterus and ovaries; urologists used it for the treatment of kidneys and ureters; general surgeons used it for the treatment of biliary-tract conditions;

thoracic surgeons used it for treating the lungs. The time-honored legitimation principles used by surgeons to distinguish themselves from others were also used to lay claim to the video laparoscopic techniques, regardless of their unique and awkward skill demands.

The general surgeons' occupational program for video laparoscopy stressed the variation inherent in human anatomy, the uniqueness of each case treated, and the necessity of developing a highly nuanced, experientially based understanding of the anatomical tract treated, regardless of treatment modality. This program argued that the intricacies of the abdominal region that general surgeons treated with conventional techniques demanded the particular and "indeterminate" skills that only they had acquired through long apprenticeship training in surgical residency. These particular craft-based skills were required to interpret highly nuanced anatomy quickly and accurately and to make sound surgical judgments on the spot with regard to the appropriate course of action. This was a time-honored logic that was used often to establish lines of demarcation among surgical specialists.

Drawing on this particularistic logic, laparoscopic general surgeons argued that success in treating surgically the upper right quadrant of the abdomen, regardless of the particular modality, demanded an intimate and detailed case-based knowledge of the peculiar structures embedded there and their relationships to one another. This was especially true for the upper right quadrant, inasmuch as this region was thought to contain "more anatomic anomalies than any other in the abdomen" (SCNA 1994a, 741). This knowledge base could only be built up over time through direct experience. Therefore, general surgeons argued that only those with prior experience in treating gallbladder disease surgically could be successful with the laparoscopic application. General surgeons argued that knowledge acquired from experience in treating other organ systems, or other regions of the anatomy, could not generalize effectively to the upper right quadrant. Technical skills in performing laparoscopy itself, although necessary, were not sufficient for treating biliary tract structures safely and effectively (ArchS 1990a; SCNA 1994a).

Moreover, 5 to 10 percent of the gallbladder cases begun laparoscopically could not be completed in that modality because of counterindications discovered during the exploratory diagnosis or during the performance of the operative procedure itself. These cases had to be converted to the open-incision modality. General surgeons argued that their particular training and experience in treating tissue through open surgery better prepared them both to choose the appropriate surgical modality for the case—either laparoscopic or open-incision—and to make the necessary conversions to the open procedure when indicated. Because of their training in the conventional technique, general surgeons argued that they were in the best position to understand and treat the complications that might arise during laparoscopy. Any division of labor that might develop between laparoscopic and conventional gallbladder surgeons would only lead to confusion and an unacceptable rate of catastrophe, because many conversions demanded on-the-spot responses.

Regardless of their technical merits, such arguments had important political ramifications for the medical profession's internal division of labor. When embraced by hospital credentialing committees, these particularistic arguments would effectively establish closure for general surgeons around all applications of the laparoscope that were extended to their conventional turf. Under the sway of these arguments, such committees closed off all nonsurgical competitors—for example, gastroenterologists and interventional radiologists—from access to the laparoscope. They also closed off access to all other surgical specialists—that is, gynecologists and perhaps some urologists—who might have developed keen laparoscopic skills but who did not have experience in conventional biliary tract surgeries. By and large, these arguments were accepted and were effective in preserving established turf divisions. Serious challenges were never mounted.

Of course, the conversion argument was not new. The same argument was used by general surgeons in the 1980s for operative endoscopy in order to prevent gastroenterologists from encroaching on surgical turf. Such arguments, however, carried little weight against the gastroenterologists, who had already established de facto control over gastrointestinal endoscopy and a precedent for doing so that was accepted as legitimate within medicine. With the laparoscopic gallbladder procedure, general surgeons moved quickly and in large numbers to establish de facto control over this new technology first. This time, general surgery's particularistic arguments for monopoly closure were heeded.

Laparoscopy as a Surgical Craft

The occupational program that surgeons used to legitimate their grip on the video laparoscope, in addition to containing the particularistic argument discussed above, involved a strong reductionist logic. This reductionist argument stressed the theoretical commonality shared in the basic cognitive approach used in all abdominal surgeries. General surgeons had used this argument, albeit with only limited success, to slow fragmentation of the craft long before the advent of laparoscopic approaches. The argument was expressed eloquently in the following surgical commentary published in 1971:

> In a very broad way there is an admirable quality of universality in surgery, regardless of the organs, systems or body cavities involved. . . . All surgery requires knowledge of the general principles of anatomy, pathology and physiology, of methods of achieving homeostasis, of avoiding infection, of eliminating dead space, and of controlling the fluid and metabolic requirements of the body before, during and after operation. Surgery requires decision and precision by the surgeon, regardless of the surgical specialty. (AnnS 1971, 331)

Surgeons embraced the logic of this time-honored argument to legitimate their grip on the laparoscope during the 1990s. They argued that laparoscopic surgery's basic principles were no different than the general principles that had undergirded the discipline of general surgery for over one hundred years. General surgeons, thus, redefined laparoscopic surgery as a technical application of surgery's most basic craft principles:

> Surgery, whether conducted by means of the laparoscopic or open route, consists of a series of logical, sequential steps, such as exposure gained by traction and countertraction, meticulous dissection, respect for surgical doctrines, operating with a plan, and having available a series of alternatives given the set of circumstances encountered. . . . Surgical principles have not changed, only the instruments with which our operations are performed have changed. (SCNA 1994c, 913, 916; see also AJS 1991n; SCNA 1994a, 742)

This reductionist logic minimized the differences between open and video techniques, defining these differences as emanating solely from technical differences in the tools used. Under the sway of this argument, the difficulties experienced with the new technique early on were the result of the initial awkwardness involved in adapting to the demands of the new instruments, not a fundamental incompatibility between the skills required to perform laparoscopy and traditional surgery. Regardless of its technical merit—and this can be questioned—this reductionist argument again favored the monopoly claims of those with experience in established conventional techniques. It devalued the claims of those who had developed laparoscopic skills but who had not yet developed specific experiential knowledge from performing surgery in the particular abdominal region in question.

In response to the very real erosion of their market turf, general surgeons embraced a radical technology of their own and developed an effective argument for extending it to other operative procedures. The latter involved the type of cognitive abstraction that Abbott discussed in *The System of Professions*. However, where Abbott linked a profession's capacity for cognitive abstraction to its ability to sustain and annex market turf in interoccupational divisions of labor, we cannot impute such causal significance to it here. The reason for this is that general surgeons employed this strategy twice. Their first attempt was a rearguard action designed to wedge into a market— the one opened up by operative endoscopy—that had already been nurtured and claimed by the gastroenterologists. Surgeons argued that for operative extensions of gastrointestinal endoscopy, their training and skills in open surgery best equipped them for safety and success. They argued that their particularistic, experientially based knowledge of the workings of the inner abdomen, their training to make quick and effective on-the-spot decisions, and their ability to react instantly to complications and perform corrective surgery if necessary would enable them to produce results superior to those of the gastroenterologists, even though the latter developed endoscopy and had honed superior skills in passing the scope and in interpreting anatomy through it.

Of course, these arguments were not strong enough to dislodge the fiber-optic endoscope from the gastroenterologists' sure grip. Gastroenterologists had established de facto control over the development of endoscopy long before the general surgeons became interested. They had developed a reputation in medicine for having honed superior endoscopic skills. And, in their hands, the shift from diagnostic to operative applications did not produce the dire consequences warned of in some of the surgical commentaries of the period. Whatever technical merits the surgeons' arguments had, they did not dissuade primary care physicians from referring patients to

gastroenterologists for operative endoscopic procedures. The limitations of the surgeons' occupational program for controlling operative
endoscopy reflected surgery's structural weakness in the downstream referral-dependent position in health care delivery. To establish the monopoly closure it needed for maintaining its market turf,
general surgeons would have to do more than embrace new technology after it had been developed by others and proffer arguments for
their monopoly closure over its application. In this case, those with
tool in hand easily beat out those embracing the rhetoric of cognitive
abstraction and reduction.

However, general surgery's second attempt was successful, and the
rhetorical strategy that surgeons used to establish monopoly closure
over operative laparoscopy was very similar to that used with operative endoscopy earlier. Surgeons argued that their particularistic
knowledge base and skills better equipped them to deliver successful outcomes with the new technology. They argued that they were
better able to manage the new technology's complications and that
their skills in the open surgical modality gave them the option of
converting to a safer procedure in the face of difficulties that arose in
5 to 10 percent of laparoscopic cases performed. Surgeons also argued
that the operative laparoscopic approaches were not radical new approaches to surgery but embodied the time-honored principles of the
surgical craft. They used these time-honored legitimation principles
to pitch their program for exclusive control over these applications
to the medical community in general and to hospital credentialing
committees in particular. Although the initial period in the development and diffusion of the new approach was quite trying, surgeons' arguments prevailed and helped to reestablish their control
over threatened market turf.

The similarities between the surgeons' rhetorical strategies for legitimating their control over the markets opened up by operative endoscopy and operative laparoscopy is striking. Essentially the same
arguments were advanced in each attempt. Although there are some
technical differences in the technologies targeted—the conversion
rate to open surgeries was much higher in operative laparoscopy than
in operative endoscopy; the laparoscopic approach enters the abdomen from the surface wall and approaches the structures treated
from the outside, while the endoscopic approach works internally
through the organ accessed—these were not the decisive factors leading to success or failure in either case.

Intraoccupational relationships and timing appear to be the more critical factors behind the success of the general surgeons' occupational program for operative laparoscopy. Here, general surgeons took de facto control over the laparoscope at the onset of the development of laparoscopic gallbladder removal. They did not propose to share this control with other specialties, as did, for example, the earlier pioneers of gastrointestinal endoscopy. General surgeons also began to develop and voice their argument for closure very quickly, long before any other competitor had established a precedent for performing the procedure. Given general surgery's downstream, referral-dependent position in health care delivery, opportune timing both in embracing a new technology and in voicing a rhetorical argument that legitimates this embrace are probably necessary conditions for establishing a jurisdiction over a new technology's application. Timing was opportune for surgeons in the case of the laparoscopic gallbladder approach and its extensions; it was not in the case of operative endoscopy.

Finally, the nature of the competitive field itself appears to have influenced the success of the surgeons' technology programs. In the case of operative endoscopy, no competitor's turf claim could be adjudicated decisively on the basis of a time-honored or legitimated precedent, for endoscopy had blurred the relevance of the divide between diagnostic, medical, and surgical treatment that had legitimated and regulated the relationship between gastroenterologists and abdominal surgeons. Gastroenterologists were not about to back off from a technology that they had spent over a decade developing, just because the general surgeons, facing tough market losses, decided to put forth a claim to it during the 1980s. Both parties believed that they had the right to perform operative procedures in the endoscopic mode. Neither respected the other's claim. Each viewed the other as an interloper. When the normative order regulating relations in a division of labor breaks down, the best bet is with those in the upstream position, whose power and resource bases are stronger.

Competitive field relations were much different in the case of operative laparoscopy. Gastroenterology's stake in the new technology was only halfhearted. It had invested heavily in other alternative approaches to treating gallbladder diseases. It was not moved to embrace the laparoscope early on because its eye was toward future applications that might obviate the need completely for gallbladder removal. Although gynecology had a strong claim to laparoscopy, it

was not in a position to ignore or forsake the particularistic-reduc-
tionist arguments that the general surgeons were advancing to stake
their claim over laparoscopic gallbladder operations. Gynecology itself had embraced similar arguments to legitimate its status claim as
an independent surgical specialty; it had used this logic to defend its
own turf against aggressive competitors. Moreover, gynecologists
were busy developing their own extensions of the video technology
to their own traditional abdominal turf—the uterus and ovaries.
Most did not desire to enter into a protracted turf war with the general surgeons. Consequently, this relational field did not engender
the same degree of fierce competition. When general surgeons staked
their claim for monopoly closure over the laparoscopic extensions to
their own abdominal turf, their potential competitors were not in a
position to mount serious counterclaims. In this case, the surgeons'
arguments for monopoly closure prevailed. The claims were respected, by and large, and were even appropriated by other surgical
specialists to protect their own endangered markets.

Notes

1. This is the typical account published in surgical journals. Horacio Asbun and
Ricardo Rossi (SCNA 1994e), however, report that a German surgeon performed the
laparoscopic procedure in September 1985 and reported it in April 1986 but that it
drew very little attention.

9

Theoretical Reflections

New technology directly impacts workplace practices, skills, interactions, and relationships, and we must always incorporate a detailed task-level focus in our accounts of technological change. To put it simply, to ignore developments at this level is to ignore most of what technology does. This task is our most basic and fundamental. However, work and occupations scholars of late have expressed a growing concern that our preoccupation with structuralist explanatory frameworks and quantitative research techniques has led us away from this essential task (see Barley 1990, 1996; Epstein 1990; Simpson 1989; Stinchcombe 1990). The detailed account of videoscopic technology's impact on surgeons' skills and work routines that I developed in chapters 1 and 2 attempted to answer these calls for more nuanced task-level accounts of work practices.

Although such accounts are the building blocks for theoretically understanding technological change, we should not lose sight of the larger market, occupational, and institutional influences that operate beyond the confines of the immediate workplace. To do so invites the derogatory label of "plant sociology" from critics of qualitative studies in the sociology of work, and this criticism is often justified. To respond to the seemingly contradictory demand for detailed accounts of developments at both the task and macro levels, we must recognize the multiple levels of social reality involved in technological change and the essential distinctiveness of the developments unfolding at each of these levels. We must recognize as well that neither the influences emanating from the workplace nor those emanating from the external environment can be accounted for adequately as a mere function of the other. Finally, we must develop conceptual tools for bridging developments from both levels into our accounts of technological change (see Barley 1990). All of this is quite difficult to do, however. By way of conclusion, I discuss how the case analysis presented here of technological change in gastrointestinal medicine might inform future research efforts attentive to these important micro-macro linkages. This present study suggests that, although often neglected, dynamics emanating from core-skill definitional processes at the intraoccupational level are critical for understanding the advent and spread of new technology. These definitional processes function to mediate the influences of both sets of forces on technological change.

Societal Dynamics

Abbott's *The System of Professions* is one of the better texts linking struggles for control over work jurisdictions among professions to larger structural and societal developments. For Abbott, the key to understanding an occupation's ability to establish control over a valued work domain lies, ultimately, in the qualities of its theoretical, or academic, knowledge base. This academic knowledge base is the foundation from which occupations' working diagnostic, inferential, and treatment classification systems develop; and professional work involves moving back and forth conceptually between the empirical problem at hand and these classification systems. For Abbott, the abstracted principles contained within a profession's academic knowledge base enable practitioners to innovate in the work arena and extend their jurisdiction to new problem domains (chaps. 2 and 3; see also Arney 1982). Professions' abilities to abstract general principles from their work practices and to apply these principles convincingly across particular problem settings, both in delivering work outcomes and in making turf claims, are the keys to their market success. As Abbott writes:

> Abstraction is the quality that sets inter-professional competition apart from competition among occupations in general. Any occupation

can obtain licensure . . . or develop an ethics code. But only a knowledge system governed by abstractions can redefine its problems and tasks, defend them from interlopers, and seize new problems. . . . Abstraction enables survival in the competitive system of professions. (1988, 8)

For Abbott, interprofessional divisions of labor tend to be unstable. Structural developments often force professions to renegotiate established work jurisdictions within these systems. The major external developments forcing system changes are technological and organizational innovations. The internal ones are expansion-minded professions and those that, for whatever reason, move out of their established jurisdictions. Such developments open and close jurisdictional spaces in the system of professions, creating vacancy chains and mobility opportunities. This consequently spurs competition among occupations holding positions there. Abbott also specifies system features that influence the intensity of this competition, such as the "connectivity" of the system's work domains and the extent to which a unifying occupational ideology regulates the professions holding positions in the system.

Abbott's theoretical framework contains many commendable features. It brings the work domain to the center of the sociology of professions. It accounts for interprofessional competition. It specifies at multiple levels many variables affecting the control of professional work. And it associates occupational developments to larger network and structural forces overlooked in past literature. However, Abbott's scheme has limitations as a framework for studying occupations in general and turf conflict in particular. My purpose here is not to dismiss the relevance of Abbott's theoretical scheme, but merely to clarify, and perhaps delimit, its scope conditions.

Abbott's central focus—interprofessional competition—may have only a circumscribed impact on occupational development. As Donald Light (1988, 205–206) has argued, we must distinguish stages in the development of professional jurisdictions. Interprofessional competition is most intense when legitimation is uncertain, typically early in the course of an occupation's development. Here, the occupation may face constant challenges from other occupations for control over its targeted work domain. Interoccupational competition is less intense, however, once the occupation in question secures a license and mandate over its work domain, especially when this is reinforced by legal sanction. Afterward, the jurisdiction takes on a locked in quality. And, interprofessional skirmishes from this point on are typically contests for control over new or peripheral tasks—not contests for control over professions' core task domains. The typical pattern with regard to occupational developments in these cases is not open turf conflict but negotiation, as the dominant occupation delegates control over peripheral task domains to weaker occupational groups within the division of labor (Larkin 1983; see also Halpern 1992).

Where occupations have locked in general jurisdictions the more significant developments are intraoccupational. Control over the task segments making up a general jurisdiction can be contested and can change, often in response to technological and organizational innovations of the type that Abbott describes. These changes can spur fierce struggles among groups operating within the occupation. At this level, however, cognitive abstraction carries much less weight in deciding the outcome of struggles than it does in the larger system of professions. We cannot simply transfer Abbott's theoretical insights here without significantly reworking them.

Abbott's own distinction between the varied arenas within which professional work jurisdictions are adjudicated is a useful starting place for developing this point. Professions secure their control over their work domains by establishing jurisdictions over them that are granted formally or informally by the state, the public, and/or the workplace organization. Abbott (chap. 3) discusses the varied nature of the claims occupations make to each of these audiences in their efforts to secure their jurisdictions. In doing so, he draws a conceptual distinction, popular among neoinstitutionalists, between a profession's institutional and technical audiences (see Meyer and Rowan 1977; Meyer and Scott 1992). From the institutional audiences—the state, the media, research foundations, and the general public—professions desire exclusive cultural authority over their work domains. Professions win support from these audiences with a rhetoric that lauds the abstracted knowledge base guiding their work performances. This abstracted knowledge base represents professions' work practices as being consistent with normative processes valued generally in society— rationalization, universalization, and the like. From the technical audiences—those with whom professionals interact directly in the workplace and in the service market—professionals mostly desire smooth processing of routines. Performance outcomes matter most, and practitioners are generally flexible in producing them. Responses to contingencies here often blur jurisdictional distinctions, however, and Abbott labels jurisdictional control at this level as "fuzzy." So long as this fuzzy reality is not acknowledged in occupations' formal representations its ambiguities tend to be tolerated and effectively managed.

Consistent with this distinction, we should conceptualize "cognitive abstraction" as having two separate and distinct components: it is a representational symbol that functions to convey information about work practices to an audience, on the one hand, and an actual component of work practices, on the other. Its importance in adjudicating work jurisdictions in the interprofessional division of labor lies primarily in its symbolic nature. Settlements between competing professions in the larger system of professions typically are hammered out at the societal level with the state and cultural institutions playing a decisive role. The cognitive abstraction of the occupation's general principles is important here because it links an occupation's claims for control over contested work domains to general modes of reasoning and modes of representing reality that society values and legitimates. Occupations' symbolic representations of themselves—their self-definitions, arguments, and justifications—are often all that decision makers have at hand when making fateful decisions. Actual work practices and their outcomes, on the other hand, have lesser importance. This "fuzzier" level of reality is difficult to know and measure reliably, and for it to weigh in on the decision making of the institutional actors governing professional jurisdictions, it must be reified and translated into accessible codes of meaning. That which makes the principles governing everyday work practices complex, contradictory, and ambiguous is not typically acknowledged or communicated to an occupation's institutional audiences. If it were, occupations' claims to status and control might be jeopardized.

The relationship between the occupational group seeking jurisdictional control over a work domain and their external audiences is different at the intraoccupational level. Generally, occupations' larger corporate bodies shield their internal conflicts from the state and the institutions representing society's interests in order to protect their jurisdictions. They close these audiences off from their internal governance processes. Consequently, groups struggling intraoccupationally for control over market turf cannot turn to them for resolution. Instead, they must turn to their own occupations' governing bodies, other interested occupational segments, and/or service recipients when making claims for jurisdictional control or in resolving disputes over market turf. As discussed more fully below, cognitive abstraction, although still important, operates much differently with these audiences. Generally, it lacks the efficacy that Abbott imputes to it, both in deciding turf contests and in directing actual work practices.

Intraoccupational Dynamics

With the recognition since the 1980s that professions are in reality diverse bodies of specialty groups that often enter into fierce competition with one another, conflict perspectives have gained some popularity in explaining occupational developments (Begun and Lippincott 1987; Bell 1986; De Santis 1980; Thomas 1994; Wilsford 1991). These perspectives typically employ a structuralist logic. Collective actions that occupational groups initiate reflect self-interests that are defined, for the most part, by these groups' structural positions in the division of labor. According to conflict perspectives, success at securing control over valued market turf comes from the power resources accruing to these structural positions.

Although the turn to conflict perspectives is certainly understandable given the historical reality, it is not entirely satisfying. First, even for functionally differentiated occupations we cannot fully embrace frameworks that stress only, or primarily, the causal significance of structural positions and the occupational interests they may generate. Simply put, turf differentiation in intraoccupational divisions of labor is not solely determined by structural position or by power resources. Its processes rarely mimic a zero-sum distribution game or an occupational variant of the Hobbesian war of all against all. Scholars studying pre-1980 specialty developments in the medical profession have stressed not open conflict among turf-hungry competitors but the role of negotiation and legitimated domination in influencing and mediating outcomes (see Bucher and Strauss 1961; Bucher 1988; Halpern 1992; Larkin 1983). Indeed, the turf conflict occurring between gastroenterology and general surgery during the 1980s and early 1990s documented above in chapter 7 was defined within the profession as exceptional and unprecedented. It represented a rare breakdown of a normative order, not anything typical or inevitable.

Second, merely shifting from theoretical frameworks that presume intraoccupational consensus to those emphasizing conflict and turf struggle does not explain fully the conflict in question. We must develop frameworks that can anticipate and explain why intraoccupational relations seem to shift back and forth between consensus and conflict. An integrated theoretical perspective that can do this will enable us to develop a deeper and more satisfying understanding of occupational dynamics. This study, by specifying critical factors that enabled an important occupational division of labor to function effectively through normative regulation, as well as those that broke it down, can serve as a prologue to such efforts.

A key to understanding intraoccupational dynamics lies in the basic insight of Everett Hughes (1971) regarding core work domains. As discussed in chapter 3 above, occupational groups embrace certain performances as more central to their occupational identities than others. Their interests in controlling their work domains draw rather narrowly around these core task performances; other tasks are not particularly valued or coveted. Indeed, workers' reactions to the performance of noncore work tasks vary from indifference to resentment. However, tasks have no inherent valuation, and definitions of a given task set's worth vary considerably from occupational group to occupational group. A task set that one occupational group defines as a necessary nuisance might be defined by another as a valued core work domain. Recognizing this tendency can provide a fuller understanding of how occupational divisions of labor self-regulate, respond to technological innovation, and break down.

Normative Regulation in Occupational Divisions of Labor

Initially, occupations mobilize their members for seizing control over a valued work domain, often in the face of intense competition from other occupations and/or occupational groups. Among other things, these mobilization efforts involve the development and conveyance of a core-skill definition that lauds the budding occupation's unique capabilities and legitimates its hold over its targeted market turf. The occupation's members embrace these definitions and use them locally to secure their positions. These definitions communicate what the occupation is all about and why its jurisdictional claims should be honored (see Bucher and Strauss 1961; Bucher 1988; Jamous and Peloille 1970; Walsh 1989).

However, as the occupation continually expands its market turf under the protection of a secured work jurisdiction, and as the complexity of its services increases with the development of new knowledge, pressures toward specialization intensify. In response, occupations often develop complex divisions of labor and means for coordinating the work activities of the various specialty groups that form within it. This type of specialization is not typically threatening to the occupation, and its processes have been well specified by those advancing the negotiation model discussed in chapter 3 (see Bucher and Strauss 1961; Bucher 1988).

The occupation's dominant segment actually encourages this type of specialization, for it embraces as its core work domain the task set around which the occupation initially mobilized. The dominant segment often devalues the new tasks that the occupation adds to its work domain as its knowledge base and service market expands. As long as it can maintain its hold over the established task set, the dominant segment is quick to delegate new task sets to others. Some members of the occupation, usually those standing far removed from its more coveted power and prestige positions, see advantages in embracing the new, and often devalued, turf. They mobilize to embrace the new task sets as their own specializations, and they tweak the occupation's core-skill definitions so as to legitimate this embrace as honorable and right. Typically, the occupation as a whole benefits from this.

Once occupations begin to develop more complex divisions of labor, coordination issues become more pressing. The extent to which these coordination issues become problematic varies by structural characteristics of the divisions of labor that emerge from these mobilization processes. James Thompson's (1967) interdependency scale provides a useful heuristic for assessing the coordination demands of these divisions of labor. Most specialties in occupational divisions of labor experience only "pooled interdependence." They handle their workloads in segmental fashion, working independently of one another. They transact directly with their clientele across a market interface. Little or no coordination among specialties is required. Systems with such characteristics experience few serious coordination problems.

Specialties experiencing "sequential," "reciprocal," or "team-level" interdependencies, however, are all dependent on other specialties during critical stages of their work processes. Of most interest to us here are sequential systems, where the output of one unit becomes the input of the subsequent unit in the workflow. Such systems make the downstream units dependent upon others for their access to clients. In occupational divisions of labor sequential interdependencies can adversely affect a specialty's market access. If upstream specialties act opportunistically, for whatever reason, downstream specialties lose markets and have little structural resources at their disposal to protect their interests.

The key to understanding the successful functioning of these divisions of labor lies in understanding how this potential for opportunism is managed, and the case of surgeons' position in the medical profession's division of labor is informative here. Surgeons have typically stood in a relationship of sequential interdependence with primary care physicians and internists. The latter screen clients for surgeons, deciding if a patient's complaint or condition merits surgical consideration. Structurally, this division of labor has placed surgeons in a dependent position, and if the medical profession's internal division of labor functioned without normative regulation, this would have gravely influenced surgeons' market access throughout its history.

However, prior to the point when the state broke the medical profession's control over its labor markets, surgery's referral-dependent position within the workflow did not seem to disadvantage its attempts to increase its market base or its status position within the profession. As discussed in chapter 4, surgery established and maintained its dominance over critical markets throughout much of the twentieth century. It did this by establishing treatment regimens that delivered valued results and by advancing claims for the superiority of these regimens that were accepted as legitimate by other occupational segments and by the profession's corporate governing bodies. The latter claims became institutionalized into scripts that upstream physicians used to process cases effectively. These scripts enabled physicians to label conditions, upon initial diagnosis, as either surgical or medical. Such scripts governed workflow between surgeons and internists sharing anatomical turf and minimized opportunism and intraoccupational conflict.

I hypothesize that such scripts generally develop among specialties in occupational divisions of labor standing in relationships of sequential interdependence. They serve the function that centralized hierarchical decision-making bodies and scheduling plans serve in hierarchical divisions of labor (see Thompson 1967). They provide ready-made answers for the simple, but critically important, question of determining who gets which case. Coordination through such scripts works normatively and cognitively rather than imperatively. Such scripts work because the actors cooperating within the division of labor believe in their efficacy. They take on a taken-for-granted quality as well.

Technological Innovation

Contradictory depictions of the relationship between technological innovation and occupational control appear in the literature. These depictions all tend to neglect the important roles that intraoccupational divisions of labor and core-skill definitions play in mediating technological developments and outcomes. Occupations, once they develop internal divisions of labor, are not homogeneous collectives. They are made up of individuals and groups with differing interests and differing core-skill definitions.

One of the most elementary and important axes of differentiation within occupations is tenure. Occupational recruits tend to identify with one another as cohorts. There will always be an established guard in intraoccupational divisions of labor that will tend to dominate the occupation's business. Members from this cohort will occupy the significant positions in the occupation's governing bodies. They will dominate local markets and will regulate the labor supply there. Subsequent cohorts will feel disadvantaged because of this and will become motivated to improve their market and status position within the occupation.

A common avenue for doing this is to embrace new technology and to create new specialties for controlling it. This essentially allows newer cohorts to establish closure over new work domains and to subject these domains to more exclusive levels of control than would otherwise be possible. It enables them to distance themselves from the established guard's dominance. It minimizes competition, and it provides opportunities for occupational mobility for new or disadvantaged members of the occupation, particularly those cohorts at the bottom of the occupation's status and market hierarchies.

Specialization is not typically resisted. When its market and status position is secure, the dominant guard willingly delegates the new technology to others. This does not usually threaten its market interests. The newer cohorts embracing the new technology typically do so in a manner that respects the legitimated dominance of the occupation's established core-skill definitions and coordination scripts. They tend to define the work problem addressed by the new technology as a special case requiring the development of special interests and skills, and they will take pains to define these interests and skills as being consistent with those lauded in the occupation's, or the specialty's, core-skill definitional frame. When they do so, their occupational programs are seldom challenged by the powers that be within the occupation.

Gastroenterology's early embrace of fiber-optic endoscopy during the 1970s illustrates this pattern well. Although gastroenterology was not a new specialty created with the introduction of the scope technology, it was a relatively new and undeveloped subspecialty of internal medicine at the time, and it embraced the new technology in a manner that was very consistent with its established core-skill definitional frame. As discussed in chapter 5, the new technology was introduced into a division of labor occupied by two major subspecialties of surgery and internal medicine—general surgery and gastroenterology. Effective scripts had developed to regulate this division of labor. These scripts labeled case conditions by their treatment types—medical or surgical. They presumed that diagnosis and treatment tasks could be performed best as separate and sequentially dependent functions. When these scripts were in place the physicians serving as gatekeepers in the profession's service delivery system—that is, those providing primary care—had little difficulty in directing a case to the proper specialist. Primary care physicians determined ownership of the case with their initial diagnosis. When either the initial diagnosis, or the frontline treatment, proved difficult or unsatisfactory, they referred the case to a gastroenterologist, who primarily functioned in the division of labor as a diagnostic consultants prior to the 1970s. Gastroenterologists used their special expertise to diagnose these difficult cases and, depending upon the diagnostic category assigned, made the decision regarding which specialty would treat the case. The scripts employed to regulate workflow in this division of labor functioned to protect the market interests of each of the specialties involved. They generated normative consensus.

As discussed in chapter 5, gastroenterologists initially embraced the fiber-optic endoscope in a manner that respected and reinforced the legitimacy of the time-honored coordination scripts regulating workflow in this division of labor. Without opposition from other specialties, gastroenterologists embraced the new technology as a diagnostic tool. This was thought to be natural and right by those working in the division of labor, since gastroenterologists had long functioned there as the master diagnosticians and had long defined their core skills in terms of their diagnostic prowess. Their initial occupational program for embracing the technology underscored this by stressing the benefits that the technology's improved diagnostic capacities would deliver for all. Because surgeons had long relied on other physicians for the initial diagnoses of their cases, they were happy to see the technology developed in the gastroenterologists' hands. They expected to reap the full benefits of this development, inasmuch as their own success rates were dependent upon diagnostic accuracy.

Whereas the gastroenterologists' initial embrace of the scope technology as a diagnostic tool functioned to neutralize cross-specialty opposition and conflict, this was not the case within the subspecialty itself. The embrace of the technology did generate opposition and conflict from within the gastroenterologists' ranks. This opposition and conflict was primarily intergenerational and cohort based. While the newer cohorts entering the subspecialty in unprecedented numbers during the 1960s and 1970s wholeheartedly embraced the new technology, the established guard watched this development with apprehension and concern. They voiced their opposition in commentaries published in the top gastroenterological journals.

The opposition did not prevail here, however. The cohorts embracing the new technology were quick to legitimate their control over it within the specialty's normative definitional frame. These newer cohorts stressed the consistency of the technology's applications with the goal most highly valued by gastroenterologists—accurate diagnosis. They argued that the new technology enhanced, rather than demeaned, the core skills long lauded in the gastroenterologists' occupational subculture.

Initially, practice seemed consistent with this rhetoric. The scope technology was used early on as a diagnostic tool, and its impressive successes were measured and quickly documented in the literature. This made it very difficult for the old guard to mount an effective countermovement in opposition to the new technology. The new technology's proponents responded forcefully to the challenges to the technology published in gastroenterological commentary, adroitly using the subspecialty's own legitimating principles in doing so. The endoscope quickly transformed gastroenterology from primarily a consulting subspecialty to a procedure-oriented subspecialty. This case trajectory is quite consistent with that specified in the negotiation model discussed in chapter 3.

Breakdown in the Normative Order

Given the technology's initial acceptance and rather smooth integration into this division of labor, how do we explain its role subsequently in breaking it down? I argue that a peculiar conjuncture of historical developments was responsible for this. First, as discussed in chapter 6, state policies undermined the medical profession's historic labor-market control. State policies encouraged the expansion of medical and surgical specialties during the 1960s and 1970s by, in essence, nationalizing and lavishly increasing the funding of medical research and development. Through its policies to increase medical school enrollments, the state also flooded physician labor markets and set off a tremendous and unprecedented wave of competition. These policies created strong market-based incentives for those physicians entering the labor market after the 1970s to both specialize and expand their market turf, even when this involved encroachment on time-honored demarcation lines. This outcome is recognized in the literature. I argued in chapters 7 and 8 that it functioned as a necessary, but not sufficient, condition for spurring the competitive developments.

However, there was more behind this turf competition. It has long been recognized that normative prescriptions mediate the influence of labor-market dynamics in occupational divisions of labor. When these prescriptions are honored, they function to control opportunism and the narrow pursuit of economic interests. However, the labor-market incentives associated with state policies regarding medical research and medical school enrollments had their impact during a period when the viability of the normative order governing the division of labor regulating gastrointestinal medicine was suddenly called into question. The normative prescriptions that were once a strong regulatory force here lost their hold. Because of this, these market effects played themselves out as they often do in un-regulated contexts.

Once gastroenterological endoscopists found that they could actually treat tissue effectively by simply threading a cutting tool through a channel built into the scope, the scripts regulating work-flow between gastroenterologists and surgeons suddenly stopped making sense. Although not its original intent, the new technology challenged surgeons' monopoly control over operative procedures. Gastroenterologists began to believe that they themselves could do a better job operating within the gastrointestinal tract for many conditions. Endoscopy did not have the same levels of trauma, morbidity, or mortality as did open surgery. For many procedures, gastroenterologists could statistically document treatment outcomes superior to that of the surgeons. The endoscope—initially introduced into this division of labor in an inconspicuous and unassuming manner—eventually developed to challenge the mystique that open surgery once held. Surgeons' special place in this division of labor, and the scripts that favored their interests there, suddenly seemed out of place.

The endoscope also challenged a fundamental assumption that normatively regulated workflow in this division of labor—the assumption that diagnosis and treatment were divisible tasks that could best be performed sequentially by different specialists. Such an assumption seemed sensible when open surgery was one of the more viable treatment options. Surgery, as a handicraft skill, demanded difficult specialized training and a large number of cases for honing and maintaining proper skill levels. Surgeons willingly specialized in this treatment modality and willingly delegated other patient care functions to others. It made little sense for them to overextend themselves as generalists when their chosen specialization demanded so much.

When gastroenterologists mobilized themselves in the 1930s and 1940s as a subspecialty of internal medicine, they filled an important and neglected niche in this division of labor. The core-skill definition with which gastroenterology mobilized new recruits emphasized diagnostic prowess, and gastroenterologists became master diagnosticians with whom primary care physicians consulted on their difficult cases. Differentiating some physicians with advanced training as primarily diagnosticians, on the one hand, and others as primarily treatment specialists, on the other, seemed sensible.

The endoscope transformed the nature of the diagnostic function and placed gastroenterologists directly at the site of diseased tissue. From this position, it made little sense to continue the rigid demarcation between diagnosis and treatment. Once cutting tools were devised for use through the endoscope, diagnosis and treatment could be accomplished in one time-bound performance. It made more sense from this point on to combine these functional tasks. Interestingly enough, those who challenged the initial efficacy of diagnostic endoscopy actually pressured gastroenterologists into taking this position. When critics began to demand that the profession judge endoscopy by its ultimate contribution to treatment outcomes, gastroenterologists were forced to move into treatment applications in defense. And they did so without abandoning the cherished core-skill definitions with which gastroenterologists had historically defined themselves and legitimated their place in the division of labor.

These developments broke the power of the scripts regulating workflow in this arena, and we must understand subsequent technological developments as unfolding in the wake of this normative breakdown. It is under this condition—one of normative breakdown—that the structural variables emphasized in conflict perspectives—those reflecting power differentials between occupational segments—have their greatest influence. In the case analysis developed above, this condition helped determine three technological outcomes: (1) gastroenterologists' embrace of operative endoscopy, (2) general surgeons' embrace of operative endoscopy, and (3) general surgeons' embrace of video laparoscopy. These developments were discussed in chapters 7 and 8.

The analyses presented above, consistent with Grace De Santis's prior study (1980), suggest that structural position in the workflow is an important determinant of the outcomes of jurisdictional contests within occupational divisions of labor. Those with direct access to clients have power advantages over those who do not. They are not as dependent on other occupational segments for their market access and can act independently and opportunistically with regard to market turf. Those in downstream referral-dependent positions have more difficulty in securing market turf. They are dependent on other gatekeeping occupational segments for their workflow, and they must act collectively to secure market turf in ways that are accepted as legitimate.

In the case study presented above, surgeons stood in the referral-dependent position. They were dependent on primary care physicians and internists for their market access. Gastroenterologists, on the other hand, typically saw patients before they went to the surgeons. As trained internists, they have historically devoted a portion of their practices to primary care. And, unlike the surgeons, their referred caseloads have tended to come from other internists who embraced a similar occupational worldview.

As discussed in chapter 7, these structural differences mattered in influencing the outcomes of the initial introduction of fiber-optic endoscopy into gastrointestinal medicine. When, with the advent of operative applications, the scope proved itself capable of becoming more than a diagnostic tool, gastroenterologists embraced it as such and used it to expand into markets where surgeons held dominance. They did this aggressively. They did this without much consideration of the consequences of such action for surgeons' livelihoods. Their advantageous structural position enabled such action. Surgeons, in contrast, could not secure their hold on this market turf, even as they somewhat clumsily embraced the fiber-optic endoscope as an operative tool. Their disadvantaged, referral-dependent position in the workflow did not provide them with ready access to the endoscopic market, and their rhetorical attempts to persuade others in the occupation to honor their market claim fell mostly on deaf ears.

So, structural location in the workflow seems to matter, and we must acknowledge its importance in our theoretical accounts of occupational development. However, the extent to which workflow position influences jurisdictional outcomes will depend on structural characteristics of the larger occupational divisions of labor themselves. Structural variables that Abbott specifies as influencing the jurisdictional outcomes of interprofessional divisions of labor will influence intraoccupational outcomes as well, such as the system's density and its units' connectivity to one another. Position in the workflow will be most influential in determining technological outcomes in systems where sequential interdependence among system units is high, less so where such interdependence is low to nonexistent.

In addition to structural position in the workflow, the timing of the specialty's embrace of new technology is critical, and this is especially the case with referral-dependent specialties. Again, general surgeons' experiences with the scope technology illustrate the significance of this variable. As discussed in chapter 7, general surgeons' attempts to legitimate their embrace of operative endoscopy came long after gastroenterologists had developed and had legitimated their hold over the diagnostic applications of this technology. Because of this unfortunate timing, and their disadvantaged structural position in the workflow, surgeons were unable to shake gastroenterologists' sure grip on the technology. Gastroenterologists had developed reputations as endoscopists, and gatekeeping physicians continued to refer their patients to them for both diagnostic and operative procedures.

As discussed in chapter 8, timing was much different in the case of video laparoscopy. Here, surgeons embraced the technology for gallbladder removal in remarkably swift fashion. The rank and file were quick to seize de facto control over this technology for the operative procedures they held. They quickly legitimated their claim for doing so before any other specialties had the opportunity to move in. Although this strategy produced some very unsavory outcomes early on, it ultimately won success.

These outcomes strongly support Glenn Gritzer's earlier arguments regarding specialization and technological innovation in medicine (1982; see also Gritzer and Arluke 1985). Gritzer contends that the development of an abstracted and esoteric knowledge base played historically only a secondary role in securing specialties' hold over their work domains. He has argued forcefully that mastery over new technology, and an ability to develop a reputation for delivering results with it, is more decisive in determining who ultimately wins jurisdiction over it (Gritzer 1982, 256; Gritzer and Arluke 1985). The importance of delivering results in determining jurisdictional outcomes reflects patients' immediate interests and, in general, the important role of clients in deciding contests for control over intraoccupational work jurisdictions (see Kronus 1976).

Indeed, service recipients constitute an audience quite different from the institutional audiences that play a vital role in legitimating the larger occupation's societal-level jurisdiction. The reified, abstracted representations of an occupation's work practices—in and of themselves—do not play as important a role in swaying the client audience. Clients in a free market are not unduly bound by a profession's formal jurisdictional control, even when this control is reinforced by a license from the state. There are few laws that prohibit prospective clients from seeking advice from whomever they please. Neither are clients unduly influenced by the eloquence of a profession's formal knowledge base, even when its expression is consistent with general societal values, as is evidenced in medicine today by the growing popularity of an expanding variety of unconventional alternatives from midwifery to acupuncture to aromatherapy. Clients' overriding concern, when in need, is for results. This concern may be the most important factor in the settlement of disputed intraoccupational task jurisdictions. As Gritzer (1982) notes, craft competence, and its emphasis upon delivering valued results, may hold the decisive advantage in intraoccupational arenas.

This is not to argue that the rhetoric of "cognitive abstraction" plays no role in jurisdictional outcomes at the intraoccupational level. Indeed, the programs that both gastroenterologists and general surgeons developed to secure jurisdictions over new technology involved such claims at every turn. Each specialty claimed that their own highly valued core knowledge base and skills easily and rightfully transferred to the new technologies in question. These claims were used to mobilize support from within each specialty and to silence or neutralize critics. The primary audience for such claims, however, were those who directly impacted market access—those in gatekeeping positions within the internal division of labor, such as the occupation's corporate bodies, hospital credentialing committees, and those working upstream in the delivery system who refer patients to the specialties in question.

Here, structural characteristics of the occupation's position in the division of labor influence jurisdictional outcomes, and these characteristics vary considerably. Those specialties, or occupational segments, establishing a direct market interface with their clients—those not dependent on referrals from other segments of the occupation—are to a great extent independent of their occupation and its corporate-level controls. Such specialties are more apt to follow their market interests, seize opportunities to expand their markets with new technologies, and less apt to seek support in doing so with official sanction from the larger occupations' corporate bodies. The rhetoric of cognitive abstraction here will probably be directed internally, used as a means to mobilize specialty members in support of a program for extending their jurisdiction to new technology. The extent to which the specialty has success with its new technology program is more dependent upon its clientele than its relationship to the larger occupation.

The case is different with referral-dependent specialties. Here, the rhetoric of cognitive abstraction is not powerful enough, in and of itself, to deliver desired results. In situations where normative regulation is weak, timing appears to be the decisive variable. The specialty must mobilize its rank and file on a massive scale, seize control over the technology in quick and decisive fashion, deliver desired results, and then make convincing rhetorical claims for controlling the technology to gatekeeping specialties and to the occupation's governing associations. All of this must be done long before competitors make a move on the technology. The critical targets of the legitimation rhetoric here are the sister specialties and occupational associations that directly control these specialties' access to client markets. Such specialties are dependent ultimately on the good will of these actors to protect their market interests in occupational divisions of labor with high levels of sequential interdependence.

The Thought Experiments

The historical conjuncture of unprecedented labor-market pressure, on the one hand, and the breakdown of the scripts normatively regulating workflow between specialties with distinctive core-skill definitions, on the other, led to the turf wars documented in chapter 7 and 8 of *Surgeons and the Scope*. The importance of this conjuncture can be highlighted by conducting the type of thought experiment that Max Weber advocated for historical sociology. What would have been the likely course of development had either of the factors in the conjuncture not materialized? What would have been the response had the specialties of gastrointestinal medicine responded to the labor-market dynamics without the concomitant development of a radical technology that challenged core-skill definitions and the normative scripts regulating those embracing them? What would have been the response had the radical technology been implemented in a labor-market context that was more effectively regulated by the occupation? Although I speculate in response to each question, my speculations are grounded in actual historical developments.

RADICAL MARKET DYNAMICS WITHOUT
TECHNOLOGICAL DISRUPTION

As discussed in chapter 6, the major specialties of the division of labor regulating gastrointestinal medicine embraced very different responses to the unprecedented labor-market dynamics that developed in response to state policies aimed at expanding the physician supply. Because of fiber-optic endoscopy's potential to open new markets for gastroenterologists, gastroenterology remained committed to a policy of expansion long after the general surgeons began to study their labor markets and advocate policies for restricting the labor supply. Without endoscopy's market promise, it seems likely that gastroenterologists, as well as other specialties, would have taken a position closer to that of the general surgeons.

As discussed in chapter 6, the general surgeons sponsored their own studies of the surgical labor market—the SOSSUS studies—and they used the findings of these studies to develop an occupational program that countered that of the state. Surgeons began to restrict entry into their residency programs and began to cut back on residency positions and programs more quickly and more effectively than did other specialties. Surgery's response to state policy might have had greater influence on other specialties had it not been for the endoscope's market-expanding promise. We can envision more cooperation between the specialties in formulating labor-market policies, tighter centralized controls over research and the expansion of research fellowships, and, in general, a more effective response to restore occupational control than that which actually developed. Surgery's own response to the labor-market threat was timely and effective. Its biggest problem was not its ability to mobilize and control its own rank and file but its inability to control the expansionary impulses of its sister specialties, most notably gastroenterology. Without the scope in hand, it is doubtful that the gastroenterologists would have taken such an aggressive approach in expanding their ranks and in crossing turf boundaries.

CONTROLLED LABOR-MARKET DYNAMICS WITH RADICAL TECHNOLOGY

The fiber-optic endoscope was not the first technology to challenge the legitimacy of the script dictating a functional separation between diagnosis and surgical treatment. Rigid endoscopes were developed around the turn of the twentieth century for accessing tissue through an orifice. Although these scopes attracted limited attention in gastrointestinal medicine, they were more widely embraced by those specializing in the treatment of more readily accessible organ systems, such as ear, nose, and throat surgeons and urologists. Although they were introduced originally as diagnostic tools, enterprising endoscopists in these fields—like those later on in gastroenterology—quickly invented mechanisms for delivering treatment through the scope.

General surgery's response to this technology, and its implicit threat to its core-skill definitions and place in the internal division of labor, was to delegate control over the technology to new specialties forming around it, even when this meant spinning off work domains that it once controlled exclusively. The new specialties developed hybrid core-skill definitions that blended components of the core-skill definitions dominant in internal medicine and surgery. They rejected the separation of diagnosis and treatment regimens as artificial, and they embraced a generalist orientation that kept the multiple functions involved in servicing their given organ systems under their unilateral control.

Had the state not flooded physicians' labor markets, such a hybrid specialization might have developed around the gastroscope. Some from the ranks of both gastroenterology and surgery were calling for such a specialization. Had this materialized, gastroenterology proper probably would have held its original place as a consulting specialty. General surgery would have retained control over its bread-and-butter surgical operations, operations that were not originally threatened by the turn to operative endoscopy. The new specialty would have taken a form similar to that of urology or gynecology, with its practitioners providing the bulk of gastrointestinal care. Like urologists and gynecologists, they would have offered primary care, diagnostic services, as well as medical and endoscopic treatments. This specialty might well have laid claim to video laparoscopy in the 1990s as well.

The deterioration of relations between gastroenterology and general surgery that had materialized by the 1980s made the cooperation necessary for developing such a specialization impractical. There were precedents for it, however, during periods when competitive labor-market dynamics were better held in check by the occupation's regulatory bodies. Such a pattern is consistent with the logic of the negotiation model discussed in chapter 3. It might have been viable under different labor-market conditions. Confining the threat of endoscopy within a separate and distinct specialty would have better protected gastroenterologists' and surgeons' core-skill definitions as well as the time-honored scripts regulating case flows within the division of labor. And the loss of markets to the new scope specialty that would have resulted would not have been as bitter or as threatening to the existing specialties if the labor market had been properly regulated by occupational control.

To conclude this section, the alternative possibilities discussed here are only meant to illustrate the factors that decisively influenced the actual course of development that materialized in the division of labor regulating gastrointestinal medicine during the 1970s and 1980s. It seems that both unprecedented labor-market developments, coupled with the breakdown of the normative scripts regulating workflow in the division of labor, led to the unprecedented turf conflict. This conjuncture of developments also influenced general surgery's unprecedented embrace of a radical technology—the video laparoscope. Had either the labor-market dynamics or the normative breakdown unfolded without the other's influence, it is unlikely that they would have led to the occupational outcomes documented in chapters 7 and 8.

Core-Skill Definitions and Work Practices

Finally, we must clarify briefly the relationship between core-skill definitions and the actual workplace practices from which they spring. Core-skill definitions are conceptual abstractions from actual everyday practice that, of necessity, gloss and simplify that reality. Core-skill definitions serve as the transmission belt bridging workplace-level reality and external reality at the intraoccupational level and beyond. Such definitions communicate to others what is essential about the work that a given occupational segment does and why their particular skills are essential to the larger work project the occupation values. Relational considerations often dictate their content. For example, I argued in chapter 7 that the emphasis in the postwar period on the cognitive bases of surgery in surgeons' self-definition was, in part, a response to the changing institutional environment within which surgeons competed for status, influence, and research funds in the medical centers.

However, as glossing abstractions, core-skill definitions typically lack the fine-grained, nitty gritty nuance required to direct work practices. As a general rule, the practice comes first. Work skills develop, adapt, and change in response to the existential reality confronted in the workplace. Skill acquisition involves actors routiniz-ing their behaviors in ways that synchronize their subjective pecu-liarities to the complexities of the immediate work environment. Such a process produces scores of particularistic stimulus-response patterns for any given task, and the particularities of these response patterns are such that they do not often transfer easily from one ac-tor to another. In work processes that involve a complex tactile di-mension these particularities are multiplied exponentially. In other words, "doing it" is much more difficult and complex than "saying what you do." And, the act of doing it is experienced differently from actor to actor. The differences between experience and account is well recognized in the sociological literature, especially in that lit-erature influenced by discourse analysis and ethnomethodology.

Consider the case of surgical work skills and the video laparo-scopic technology discussed above. In the rhetoric of the general sur-geons, the adoption of this technology involved a process that Abbott refers to as "simple reduction" in *The System of Professions*. The core-skills involved in the surgeons' traditional work performance and that involved in the performance of the new laparoscopic surgery were one and the same. The general abstracted principles were the same, the steps were for all practical purposes the same, and the stock of knowledge involved in the performance was the same. At the level of definition and rhetoric the primary difference between the performances was in simply learning how to manipulate new tools.

At the level of the behavioral performance, however, the differ-ences between the work practices demanded for success by these dif-ferent modalities were stark—stark enough for informants to suggest that many of those trained and facile with the traditional techniques could not adequately adjust to the demands of the new technology. The reasons for this were documented in chapters 1 and 2 above. The new surgical modality demanded very different behaviors from the individual surgeon than the old one did. The basic movements in-volved in task performances, the hand-eye coordination required for guiding the performance, the basic spatial positioning of tools and personnel, and, most importantly, the manner in which the surgeon and the surgical assistants coordinated their efforts with one another were all very different. Although these types of nuanced, fine-grained components of behavioral performance rarely are expressed in core-skill definitions, and although they are most likely taken for granted and seldom discussed, theorized, or accounted outside of the immediate operating-room context after a surgeon's initial training, they are vital to the performance's success. As documented in chapter 8, surgery's initial failure to adjust and account for these differences adequately almost delegitimated the specialty's claims for monopoly closure over the applications of video laparoscopy that extended into their traditional turf, such as gallbladder removal.

As the case of general surgery's embrace of the video laparoscopic technology suggests, core-skill definitions are nothing more than abstracted representations of selected behaviors rooted in the particularistic details of everyday work performances. I believe it is a mistake to view core-skill definitions, in and of themselves, as effectively directing work practices or shaping their particularistic contours. It is not the abstracted principles that enable an occupational group to move from one technology to another but the more microlevel, seldom-accounted-for adjustments to sedimented behavioral routines. The outcomes of these adjustments must be accounted for in our scholarly reports of technological change, and chapters 1 and 2 did this for general surgery. Although such adjustments are not institutionalized at the occupational level, their success is far from automatic with radical new technology. They may lead to unintended and unanticipated developmental courses.

Contemporary developments have led some scholars to suggest a more prominent role for occupational divisions of labor in the new economy. In stark contrast to the hierarchical divisions of labor that have dominated work organization throughout the twentieth century, occupational divisions of labor are largely decentralized structures that pass decision-making authority to the producers. Contemporary developments have sparked renewed interest in how these types of systems organize, coordinate their work activities, and respond to technological and organizational innovations. It behooves us to match the historical changes we are witnessing with a new wave of conceptual refinement and development. By sensitizing us to the importance of core-skill definitional processes and their concomitant intraoccupational developments in influencing technological change outcomes, *Surgeons and the Scope* makes a contribution to this larger academic project. It is my hope that, with critique, revision, and reformulation, the conceptualizations presented and developed here will have general utility for understanding technological change in occupational divisions of labor.

Methodological Appendix

Analyses of the workplace outcomes of technological change must begin with detailed understandings of the task domains affected. Our understanding must cut deeper than the stereotypical views we often carry with us into the research setting about the nature of the work in question. We should produce both an in-depth description of typical work tasks and an account of their meanings to those enacting them. This should be the necessary first step of any workplace analysis. Qualitative approaches—participant observation and depth interviewing—are best, and probably necessary, for achieving this.

To acquire this level of familiarity with surgical work, I conducted qualitative interviews during 1994 and 1995 with thirty-seven informants who were using either endoscopic, laparoscopic, or laser instruments in surgical or therapeutic procedures in six communities from a region of upstate New York. I contacted those who listed one of these procedures in the classified pages of the phone book by letter and then phone. Following the invitation of informants, I made direct observations of two videoscopic procedures.

The interview guide was loosely structured to elicit comparisons between the new procedures and conventional techniques in terms of the work skills, work routines, and work relationships involved. The new technology was a recent innovation. Informants typically could produce vivid and thoughtful comparisons between the practices and skills the new technology demanded and those demanded by conventional procedures. The interview guide was followed loosely. Once respondents began discussing a given procedure, I probed extensively for elaboration. Most of the questions I asked during the interviews, in fact, followed topics brought up in respondents' accounts of their technological experiences. I tape-recorded and personally transcribed each interview soon after the event. Constant reviews of the transcripts were made during all stages of data collection. Ideas and hypotheses were developed, tested, discarded, and refined in process (see Glaser and Strauss 1967).

My initial research plan, influenced by media reports, focused on the laser component of "minimally invasive" surgeries. "Laser surgery" was the buzzword associated with many of the newer laparoscopic approaches—the label often used in the titles of popular magazine articles. And, initially, I found the thought of the laser replacing surgeons' skilled hands intriguing and, given my off-hand impression of surgeons' workplace control, rather puzzling. How could surgeons embrace such a technology?

My very first informant gave me an intriguing answer to this. This informant defined the laser procedure in which his group had invested as a low-skilled procedure. The informant was quick to differentiate the nature of the skills involved in "true" surgeries from those involved in the laser procedure. His laser was purchased for a very specialized procedure, and the group was in the process of delegating control over the procedure to their nurses, thereby freeing up their time for the conventional surgeries they performed. In sharp contrast to this case, however, my second informant talked up the laser in a very different way, emphasizing the new skills its use demanded. This informant's ego seemed to be heavily invested in the technology, and he seemed to define his proficiency with it as an important facet of his professional identity. These accounts did not mesh well. Each informant treated surface tissue, and neither used the video technology.

My third informant actually had conducted surgical procedures using the video technology, and it became apparent to me from this informant's account that it was the video equipment, and not so much the energy source used, that profoundly changed surgeons' operating routines. My interviews with all subsequent informants with experience with the videoscope confirmed this emphasis, and one lesson I learned was that surgeons did not define the manual task of cutting tissue per se as a particularly difficult or virtuous activity. Although it was certainly important, interpreting anatomy and making proper judgments on the basis of these interpretations were deemed much more vital to success. Skills developing around these critical activities were those that distinguished "true" surgeons from those with lesser virtue. The demands of the videoscopic technology—working through small ports, interpreting and directing the surgical process from an image projected from a miniaturized camera onto television screens, and manipulating long instruments outside of the closed abdomen—made these critical tasks more difficult to accomplish. These are the factors my informants talked up as significant, and I shifted my research focus accordingly.

I tried to pinpoint the specific workplace effects of the various components of the new technology—that is, the video system, the various energy sources, and the technology's peculiar mode of access. Although intentions, definitions, cultural influences, and the like are all important in influencing workplace outcomes, technology itself often asserts an obdurate impact of its own (see Adler 1992; Barley 1986, 1990; Clark et al. 1988; Noble 1984, chap. 11). It often stands as a force to be reckoned with on terms not entirely defined or anticipated by its users or designers. To distinguish these effects from others, I sought out informants experienced with varying components of the technology from across specialty areas (gynecologists, general surgeons, urologists, gastroenterologists, and specialty surgeons), communities (six communities from upstate New York), and training locales (residency programs in, and outside of, a regional medical center).

Most importantly, my informants had varied experiences with the components of the technology itself. Although most informants removed structures through the scope with the video camera and television monitors, some only performed simpler procedures. One informant, for example, did not use the video system. He conducted procedures while peering through an eyepiece attached to the base of the scope. This practice was common prior to the advent of the video system. Some informants performed endoscopic procedures but not the sophisticated laparoscopic procedures upon which this book focuses most intensively. And two informants—my first two—only used lasers. The accounts from those informants in chapters 1 and 2 who did not perform the full range of videoscopic procedures served as contrast cases to the accounts from those who did. They helped me pinpoint the various effects of the new technology's components.

Given the diversity in my sample, there was surprisingly little variation in my informants' actual accounts of the skill demands of the new technology that could not be attributed to differences in its technical components. What it was like, for instance, to guide instruments from the image on the screen through the scope or a trocar port was described similarly whether the informant was a gynecologists, general surgeon, urologist, or gastroenterologist. I take this similarity as support for a claim that this technology itself generated distinctive demands on those using it, regardless of their specialty or personal backgrounds. I used the interview information I collected to construct a general portrayal of the videoscopic technology's impact on surgical routines.

The questions of why this technology was wheeled into the operating room in the first place and why it spread throughout surgery have to be addressed as well. To do this, I had to shift my focus from the more micro level—what folks did with their minds and hands in the operating room—to a more macro level. I had to understand how surgeons' operating-room definitions and practices fit into the larger division of labor governing specialty relations. My focus also had to become historical, inasmuch as these larger relations developed and changed over time, and this developmental process intertwined with those involved in technological change. The interview data did not provide sufficient information for this.

To speak informatively on these issues, I needed information regarding the larger division of labor, who the most relevant players were in gastrointestinal medicine and how they related to one another. I also needed information regarding how these specialties defined their relationship to the scope technology, how the technology related to their self-defined core tasks and skills, and how their embrace of the technology impacted their relationships with other specialties. The primary information I collected for this was archival—information from articles, editorials, and commentary published in medical specialty journals. I used the *Index Medicus*, an exhaustive index to medical literature, to locate texts published from 1960 to 1995. The specialty journals proved vital to my research aims, because they were the way specialty associations communicated with their rank and file.

Although the interview information served as the primary source for my descriptive account of the videoscopic technology's impact on operating-room routines, it also grounded the historical research. After conducting thirty-seven interviews, I had a much better understanding of the surgical process and the technology affecting it, and this understanding provided a background framework for searching for, and interpreting, the archival information. In turn, the archival notes were coded in the same way as the interview transcripts, and they were analyzed to check for consistency and inconsistency in the interview data (on triangulating this type of data, see Zetka and Walsh 1994).

Works Cited

General

Abbott, Andrew D. 1988. *The System of Professions: An Essay on the Division of Expert Labor.* Chicago: University of Chicago Press.

Adler, Paul S., ed. 1992. *Technology and the Future of Work.* New York: Oxford University Press.

Altman, Stuart H. 1984. "The Growing Physician Surplus: Will It Benefit or Bankrupt the U.S. Health System?" In *The Coming Physician Surplus: In Search of a Policy,* edited by Eli Ginzberg and Miriam Ostow, 9–36. Totawa, N.J.: Rowman and Allanheld.

Arney, William R. 1982. *Power and the Profession of Obstetrics.* Chicago: University of Chicago Press.

Atkinson, Paul. 1971. "Professional Segmentation and Students' Experience in a Scottish Medical School." *Scottish Journal of Sociology* 2: 71–85.

———. 1981. *The Clinical Experience: The Construction and Reconstruction of Medical Reality.* Westmead, England: Gower.

Atkinson, Paul, Margaret Reid, and Peter Sheldrake. 1977. "Medical Mystique." *Sociology of Work and Occupations* 4: 243–80.

Baer, William C. 1986. "Expertise and Professional Standards." *Work and Occupations* 13: 532–52.

Barley, Stephen R. 1986. "Technology as an Occasion for Structuring: Evidence from Observations of CT Scanners and the Social Order of Radiology Departments." *Administrative Science Quarterly* 31: 78–108.

———. 1990. "The Alignment of Technology and Structure through Roles and Networks." *Administrative Science Quarterly* 35: 61–103.

———. 1996. "Technicians in the Workplace: Ethnographic Evidence for Bringing Work into Organization Studies." *Administrative Science Quarterly* 41: 404–41.

Becker, Howard S., Blanche Geer, Everett C. Hughes, and Anselm L. Strauss.

1961. *Boys in White: Student Culture in Medical School.* Chicago: University of Chicago Press.

Begun, James W., and Ronald C. Lippincott. 1987. "The Origins and Resolution of Interoccupational Conflict." *Work and Occupations* 14: 368–86.

Bell, Susan E. 1986. "A New Model of Medical Technology Development: A Case Study of DES." *Research in the Sociology of Health Care* 4: 1–32.

Berlant, Jeffrey L. 1975. *Profession and Monopoly: A Study of Medicine in the United States and Great Britain.* Berkeley: University of California Press.

Boreham, Paul. 1983. "Indetermination: Professional Knowledge, Organization, and Control." *Sociological Review* 31: 693–718.

Bosk, Charles L. 1979. *Forgive and Remember: Managing Medical Failure.* Chicago: University of Chicago Press.

Braverman, Harry. 1974. *Labor and Monopoly Capital: The Degradation of Work in the Twentieth Century.* New York: Monthly Review.

Bucher, Rue. 1962. "Pathology: The Study of Social Movements in a Profession." *Social Problems* 10: 40–51.

———. 1988. "On the Natural History of Health Care Occupations." *Work and Occupations* 15: 131–47.

Bucher, Rue, and Joan G. Stelling. 1977. *Becoming Professional.* Beverly Hills, Calif.: Sage.

Bucher, Rue, and Anselm L. Strauss. 1961. "Professions in Process." *American Journal of Sociology* 66: 325–34.

Carlton, Wendy. 1978. *"In Our Professional Opinion . . .": The Primacy of Clinical Judgment over Moral Choice.* Notre Dame, Ind.: University of Notre Dame Press.

Carr-Saunders, Alexander M., and Paul A. Wilson. 1933. *The Professions.* Oxford: Clarendon.

Cartwright, Frederick F. 1967. *The Development of Modern Surgery.* New York: Crowell.

Cassell, Joan. 1991. *Expected Miracles: Surgeons at Work.* Philadelphia: Temple University Press.

Chang, Sophia W., and Harold S. Luft. 1991. "Reimbursement and the Dynamics of Surgical Procedure Innovation." In *The Changing Economics of Medical Technology*, edited by Annetine C. Gelijns and Ethan A. Halm, 96–122. Washington: National Academy Press.

Child, John, and Janet Fulk. 1982. "Maintenance of Occupational Control: The Case of Professions." *Work and Occupations* 9: 155–92.

Clark, Jon, Ian McLoughlin, Howard Rose, and Robin King. 1988. *The Process of Technological Change: New Technology and Social Choice in the Workplace.* Cambridge: Cambridge University Press.

Cooper, Theodore, and Nicholas A. Olimpio. 1980. "Medical Education." In *Regulating Health Care: The Struggle for Control*, edited by Arthur Levin, 32–44. New York: Academy of Political Science.

Coser, Rose Laub. 1958. "Authority and Decision-Making in a Hospital: A Comparative Analysis." *American Sociological Review* 23: 56–64.

———. 1962. *Life in the Ward.* East Lansing: Michigan State University Press.

De Santis, Grace. 1980. "Realms of Expertise: A View from within the Medical Profession." *Research in the Sociology of Health Care* 1: 179–236.

Elliott, Philip. 1972. *The Sociology of Professions*. New York: Herder and Herder.

Epstein, Cynthia Fuchs. 1990. "The Cultural Perspective and the Study of Work." In *The Nature of Work: Sociological Perspectives*, edited by Kai Erikson and Steven Peter Vallas, 88–98. New Haven: Yale University Press.

Esland, Geoff. 1980. "Professions and Professionalism." In *The Politics of Work and Occupations*, edited by Geoff Esland and Graeme Salaman, 213–50. Milton Keynes, England: Open University Press.

Fein, Rashi, and Gerald I. Weber. 1971. *Financing Medical Education: An Analysis of Alternative Policies and Mechanisms*. New York: McGraw-Hill.

Feldstein, Paul J. 1977. *Health Associations and the Demand for Legislation: The Political Economy of Health*. Cambridge, Mass.: Ballinger.

Fox, Renée C. 1957. "Training for Uncertainty." In *The Student-Physician: Introductory Studies in the Sociology of Medical Education*, edited by Robert K. Merton, George G. Reader, and Patricia L. Kendall, 207–44. Cambridge: Harvard University Press.

——. 1989. *The Sociology of Medicine: A Participant Observer's View*. Englewood Cliffs, N.J.: Prentice-Hall.

Fox, Renée C., and Judith P. Swazey. 1978. *The Courage to Fail: A Social View of Organ Transplants and Dialysis*. 2nd ed. Chicago: University of Chicago Press.

Freidson, Eliot. 1970a. *Professional Dominance: The Social Structure of Medical Care*. New York: Atherton.

——. 1970b. *Profession of Medicine: A Study of the Sociology of Applied Knowledge*. New York: Dodd, Mead.

——. 1984. "The Changing Nature of Professional Control." *Annual Review of Sociology* 10: 1–20.

——. 1986. *Professional Powers: A Study of the Institutionalization of Formal Knowledge*. Chicago: University of Chicago Press.

——. 1994. *Professionalism Reborn: Theory, Prophecy, and Policy*. Chicago: University of Chicago Press.

——. 2001. *Professionalism: The Third Logic*. University of Chicago Press.

Galaskiewicz, Joseph. 1985. "Professional Networks and the Institutionalization of a Single Mind-Set." *American Sociological Review* 50: 639–58.

Ginzberg, Eli. 1984. "Conference Summary, the Expanding Physician Supply: Policy Options." In *The Coming Physician Surplus: In Search of a Policy*, edited by Eli Ginzberg and Miriam Ostow, 1–8. Totawa, N.J.: Rowman and Allanheld.

——, ed. 1986. *From Physician Shortage to Patient Shortage: The Uncertain Future of Medical Practice*. Boulder, Colo.: Westview.

——. 1990. *The Medical Triangle: Physicians, Politicians, and the Public*. Cambridge: Harvard University Press.

Ginzberg, Eli, Edward Brann, Dale Hiestand, and Miriam Ostow. 1981. "The Expanding Physician Supply and Health Policy." *Milbank Quarterly* 59: 508–41.

Glaser, Barney G., and Anselm L. Strauss. 1967. *The Discovery of Grounded Theory: Strategies for Qualitative Research*. Chicago: Aldine.

Glaser, Robert J. 1966. "The Teaching Hospital and the Medical School." In *The*

Teaching Hospital: Evolution and Contemporary Issues, edited by John H. Knowles, 7–37. Cambridge: Harvard University Press.

Gritzer, Glenn. 1982. "Occupational Specialization in Medicine: Knowledge and Market Explanations." *Research in the Sociology of Health Care* 2: 251–83.

Gritzer, Glenn, and Arnold Arluke. 1985. *The Making of Rehabilitation: A Political Economy of Medical Specialization, 1890–1980*. Berkeley: University of California Press.

Halm, Ethan A., and Annetine Gelijns. 1991. "An Introduction to the Changing Economics of Technological Innovation in Medicine." In *The Changing Economics of Medical Technology*, edited by Annetine C. Gelijns and Ethan A. Halm, 1–20. Washington: National Academy Press.

Halpern, Sydney A. 1992. "Dynamics of Professional Control: Internal Coalitions and Crossprofessional Boundaries." *American Journal of Sociology* 97: 994–1021.

Hiestand, Dale L. 1984. "Medical Residencies in a Period of Expanding Physician Supply." In *The Coming Physician Surplus: In Search of a Policy*, edited by Eli Ginzberg and Miriam Ostow, 69–82. Totawa, N.J.: Rowman and Allanheld.

Hodson, Randy. 1988. "Good Jobs and Bad Management: How New Problems Evoke Old Solutions in High-Tech Settings." In *Industries, Firms, and Jobs: Sociological and Economic Approaches*, edited by George Farkas and Paula England, 247–79. New York: Plenum.

Hoff, Timothy J., and David P. McCaffrey. 1996. "Adapting, Resisting, and Negotiating: How Physicians Cope with Organizational and Economic Change." *Work and Occupations* 23: 165–89.

Hoffman, Lily M. 1989. *The Politics of Knowledge: Activist Movements in Medicine and Planning*. Albany: State University of New York Press.

Hollingsworth, J. Rogers. 1986. *A Political Economy of Medicine: Great Britain and the United States*. Baltimore, Md.: Johns Hopkins University Press.

Hughes, Everett C. 1971. *The Sociological Eye: Selected Papers*. Chicago: Aldine-Atherton.

Jamous, H., and B. Peloille. 1970. "Professions or Self-Perpetuating Systems? Changes in the French University-Hospital System." In *Professions and Professionalization*, edited by J. A. Jackson, 109–52. Cambridge: Cambridge University Press.

Johnson, Terence J. 1972. *Professions and Power*. London: Macmillan.

Katz, Pearl. 1981. "Ritual in the Operating Room." *Ethnology* 20: 335–50.

———. 1985. "How Surgeons Make Decisions." In *Physicians of Western Medicine: Anthropological Approaches to Theory and Practice*, edited by Robert A. Hahn and Atwood D. Gaines, 155–75. Boston: D. Reidel.

Kendall, Patricia L. 1963. "The Learning Environments of Hospitals." In *The Hospital in Modern Society*, edited by Eliot Freidson, 195–230. Glencoe, Ill.: Free Press.

Knafl, Kathleen, and Gary Burkett. 1975. "Professional Socialization in a Surgical Specialty: Acquiring Medical Judgment." *Social Science and Medicine* 9: 397–404.

Kronus, Carol L. 1976. "Occupational versus Organizational Influences on Reference Group Identification." *Work and Occupations* 3: 303–30.

Larkin, Gerald V. 1983. *Occupational Monopoly and Modern Medicine*. London: Tavistock.

Larson, Magali Sarfatti. 1977. *The Rise of Professionalism: A Sociological Analysis*. Berkeley: University of California Press.

Lawton, Stephan, and JoAnne Glisson. 1977. "Congressional Deliberations: A Commentary." In *Deliberations and Compromise: The Health Professions Educational Assistance Act of 1976*, edited by Lauren LeRoy and Philip R. Lee. 1–19. Cambridge, Mass.: Ballinger.

LeRoy, Lauren, and Philip R. Lee, eds. 1977. *Deliberations and Compromise: The Health Professions Educational Assistance Act of 1976*. Cambridge, Mass.: Ballinger.

Light, Donald W. 1986. "Surplus versus Cost Containment: The Changing Context for Health Providers." In *Applications of Social Science to Clinical Medicine and Health Policy*, edited by Linda H. Aiken and David Mechanic, 519–42. New Brunswick, N.J.: Rutgers University Press.

——. 1988. "Turf Battles and the Theory of Professional Dominance." *Research in the Sociology of Health Care* 7: 203–25.

Litman, Theodor J. 1991. "Chronology and Capsule Highlights of the Major Historical and Political Milestones in the Evolutionary Involvement of Government in Health and Health Care in the United States." In *Health Politics and Policy*, 2nd ed., edited by Theodor J. Litman and Leonard S. Robins, 395–411. Albany, N.Y.: Delmar Press.

Marsden, Lorna R. 1977. "Power within a Profession: Medicine in Ontario." *Sociology of Work and Occupations* 4: 3–26.

McPherson, Klim, P. M. Strong, Arnold Epstein, and Lesley Jones. 1981. "Regional Variations in the Use of Common Surgical Procedures: Within and between England and Wales, Canada and the United States of America." *Social Science and Medicine* 15A: 273–88.

Meyer, John W., and Brian Rowan. 1977. "Institutionalized Organizations: Formal Structure as Myth and Ceremony." *American Journal of Sociology* 83: 340–63.

Meyer, John W., and W. Richard Scott. 1992. *Organizational Environments: Ritual and Rationality*. Newbury Park, Calif.: Sage.

Millman, Michael L. 1980. *Politics and the Expanding Physician Supply*. Montclair, N.J.: Allanheld, Osmun.

Morris, Robert T. 1935. *Fifty Years a Surgeon*. New York: Dutton.

Mumford, Emily. 1970. *Interns: From Students to Physicians*. Cambridge: Harvard University Press.

Noble, David F. 1984. *Forces of Production: A Social History of Industrial Automation*. New York: Knopf.

Nolen, William A. 1970. *The Making of a Surgeon*. New York: Random House.

Perrow, Charles. 1984. *Normal Accidents: Living with High-Risk Technologies*. New York: Basic Books.

——. 1986. *Complex Organizations: A Critical Essay*. 3rd ed. New York: McGraw-Hill.

Pinch, Trevor, H. M. Collins, and Larry Carbone. 1997. "Cutting Up Skills: Estimating Difficulty as an Element of Surgical and Other Abilities." In *Between Craft and Science: Technical Work in U.S. Settings*, edited by Stephen R. Barley and Julian E. Orr, 101–12. Ithaca: Cornell University Press.

Rosengren, William R., and Spencer DeVault. 1963. "The Sociology of Time and Space in an Obstetrical Hospital." In *The Hospital in Modern Society*, edited by Eliot Freidson, 266–92. Glencoe, Ill.: Free Press.

Russell, Paul S. 1966. "Surgery in a Time of Change." In *The Teaching Hospital: Evolution and Contemporary Issues*, edited by John H. Knowles, 38–65. Cambridge: Harvard University Press.

Schneller, Eugene S. 1978. *The Physician's Assistant: Innovation in the Medical Division of Labor*. Lexington, Mass.: Lexington.

Shaiken, Harley. 1984. *Work Transformed: Automation and Labor in the Computer Age*. New York: Holt, Rinehart, and Winston.

Shortell, Stephen M. 1973. "Patterns of Referral among Internists in Private Practice: A Social Exchange Model." *Journal of Health and Social Behavior* 14: 335–48.

Shryock, Richard H. 1979 [1974]. *The Development of Modern Medicine: An Interpretation of the Social and Scientific Factors Involved*. Madison: University of Wisconsin Press.

Simpson, Ida Harper. 1989. "The Sociology of Work: Where Have the Workers Gone?" *Social Forces* 67: 563–81.

Simpson, Richard L. 1985. "Social Control of Occupations and Work." *Annual Review of Sociology* 11: 415–36.

Starr, Paul. 1982. *The Social Transformation of American Medicine*. New York: Basic Books.

Stevens, Rosemary. 1971. *American Medicine and the Public Interest*. New Haven: Yale University Press.

——. 1986. "The Changing Hospital." In *Applications of Social Science to Clinical Medicine and Health Policy*, edited by Linda H. Aiken and David Mechanic, 80–99. New Brunswick, N.J.: Rutgers University Press.

Stinchcombe, Arthur L. 1959. "Bureaucratic and Craft Administration of Production: A Comparative Study." *Administrative Science Quarterly* 4: 168–87.

——. 1990. "Work Institutions and the Sociology of Everyday Life." In *The Nature of Work: Sociological Perspectives*, edited by Kai Erickson and Steven Peter Vallas, 99–116. New Haven: Yale University Press.

Strauss, Anslem, Leonard Schatzman, Rue Bucher, Danuta Ehrlich, and Melvin Sabshin. 1964. *Psychiatric Ideologies and Institutions*. Glencoe, Ill.: Free Press.

Thomas, Robert J. 1994. *What Machines Can't Do: Politics and Technology in the Industrial Enterprise*. Berkeley: University of California Press.

Thompson, James D. 1967. *Organizations in Action: Social Science Bases of Administrative Theory*. New York: McGraw-Hill.

Trice, Harrison M. 1993. *Occupational Subcultures in the Workplace*. Ithaca, N.Y.: ILR Press.

Van Maanen, John, and Stephen R. Barley. 1984. "Occupational Communities:

Culture and Control in Organizations." *Research in Organizational Behavior* 6: 287–365.

Wallace, Michael. 1989. "Brave New Workplace: Technology and Work in the New Economy." *Work and Occupations* 16: 363–92.

Walsh, John P. 1989. "Technological Change and the Division of Labor: The Case of Retail Meatcutters." *Work and Occupations* 16: 165–83.

Wechsler, Henry. 1976. *Handbook of Medical Specialties*. New York: Human Science.

Wilsford, David. 1991. *Doctors and the State: The Politics of Health Care in France and the United States*. Durham, N.C.: Duke University Press.

Wilson, Robert N. 1954. "Teamwork in the Operating Room." *Human Organization* 12: 9–14.

Zetka, James R., Jr., and John P. Walsh. 1994. "A Qualitative Protocol for Studying Technological Change in the Labor Process." *Bulletin de methodologie sociologique* 45: 37–73.

Medical Journal and Newspaper References

(AIM) ANNALS OF INTERNAL MEDICINE

1993a. On endoscopic training and procedural competence, by John Baillie and William J. Ravich, vol. 118, 73–74.

1993b. Objective evaluation of endoscopy skills during training, by Oliver W. Cass, Martin L. Freeman, Craig J. Peine, Richard T. Zera, and Gerald R. Onstad, vol. 118, 40–44.

(AJG) AMERICAN JOURNAL OF GASTROENTEROLOGY

1962. Laparoscopy (peritoneoscopy) and guided liver biopsy, II, by Gustav A. Uhlich and William S. Haubrich, vol. 38, 313–21.

1977. Primary sclerosing cholangitis, by John Ackert and Hillel Tobias, vol. 68, 498–500.

1978a. Delayed ("blow-out") perforation of sigmoid following diagnostic colonoscopy, by Angelo E. Dagradi, Mary E. Norris, and Zelman G. Weingarten, vol. 70, 317–20.

1978b. Presidential address, by F. Warren Nugent, vol. 69, 141–43.

1978c. Recent advances in gastrointestinal endoscopy, by L. Demling, vol. 69, 533–43.

1979. The training of a gastrointestinal endoscopist, by Angelo E. Dagradi, vol. 71, 224–28.

1981. Guidelines for training in gastroenterology, by Franz Goldstein, Arvey I. Rogers, and Burton I. Korelitz, vol. 76, 235–38.

1983a. The first fifty years—a history of evolution of the American College of Gastroenterology as a society for clinical gastroenterology, by David A. Dreiling, vol. 78, 138–39.

1983b. Parsnips and pomegranates—training in gastroenterology then and now, by Howard M. Spiro, vol. 78, 57–62.

1984a. The case for *surgical* training in gastrointestinal endoscopy, by John S. Kukora, Charles P. Clericuzio, and Thomas L. Dent, vol. 79, 907–9.

1984b. Current status of endoscopic sphincterotomy, by Stephen E. Silvis, vol. 79, 731–33.

1984c. Lasers and gastroenterology, by David Fleischer, vol. 79, 406–15.

1984d. Percutaneous endoscopic jejunostomy, by Jeffrey L. Ponsky and Ami Aszodi, vol. 79, 113–16.

1984e. Who said surgeons had to be trained in gastrointestinal endoscopy? by James L. Achord, vol. 79, 322–23.

1985a. To the editor, by James L. Achord, vol. 80, 233.

1985b. Surgeons and gastrointestinal endoscopy, by William Silen, vol. 80, 232.

1985c. Who should do gastrointestinal endoscopy? by Angelo E. Dagradi, vol. 80, 658.

1986a. An evaluation of performance after informal training in endoscopic retrograde sphincterotomy, by J. T. Frakes, vol. 81, 512–15.

1986b. Gastroenterology and the American college, by Walter H. Jacobs, vol. 81, 213–17.

1986c. When push comes to shove, by R.A. Kozarek, T. J. Ball, and J. A. Ryan Jr., vol. 81, 642–46.

1987a. The credentialing process, by James L. Achord, vol. 82, 1064–5.

1987b. Endoscopy, obstructive jaundice, and DRGs, by Jerome H. Siegel, Melvin Schapiro, and Rollin W. Hughes Jr., vol. 82, 173–74.

1987c. Evaluation of procedural skills in gastroenterologists, by John A. Benson Jr. and Sidney Cohen, vol. 82, 669.

1987d. Medical education and gastrointestinal fellowship training, by Martin H. Floch, vol. 82, 880–81.

1987e. The 1986 American College of Gastroenterology membership survey, by Chesley Hines Jr., vol. 82, 1004–11.

1988a. Alternatives to cholecystectomy and common duct exploration, by David S. Zimmon, vol. 83, 1272–3.

1988b. Interventional endoscopy in the pancreatobiliary tree, by J. F. Dowsett, D. Vaira, A. Polydorou, R. O. G. Russell, and P. R. Salmon, vol. 83, 1328–36.

1989. The community hospital gastroenterologist, by Melvin Schapiro, vol. 84, 229–32.

1990. Retained bile duct stones, by Peter B. Cotton, vol. 85, 1075–8.

1991. A study of gastroenterologists in the United States, by Anne Elixhauser, Peter McMenamin, and Christina Witsberger, vol. 86, 406–11.

1992. Up close and personal, by Arvey I. Rogers, vol. 87, 1542–6.

1993a. The accuracy of endoscopic estimates, by Jerome D. Waye, vol. 88, 483–84.

1993b. Are endoscopic measurements of colonic polyps reliable? by M. Brian Fennerty, Jonelle Davidson, Scott S. Emerson, Richard E. Sampliner, Lee J. Hixson, and Harinder S. Garewal, vol. 88, 496–500.

1993c. Laparoscopic cholecystectomy, by Scott M. Wiesen, Stephen W. Unger, Jamie S. Barkin, David S. Edelman, James S. Scott, and Harold M. Unger, vol. 88, 334–37.

1993d. Laparoscopic cholescystectomy for acute cholecystitis, by Robert J. Fitzgibbons, Jr. vol. 88, 330–31.

1993e. A question of quality, by Sarkis J. Chobanian, Arvey Rogers, and Lawrence J. Brandt, vol. 88, 329–30.

(AJOG) AMERICAN JOURNAL OF OBSTETRICS AND GYNECOLOGY

1970. Recent experience with diagnostic and surgical laparoscopy, by Robert S. Neuwirth, vol. 106, 119–21.

1992. Infertility and endometriosis, by Norman F. Gant, vol. 166, 1072–81.

1993a. Discussion, by Dennis J. Lutz, vol. 168, 1698–9.

1993b. Operative laparoscopy, by Yona Tadir and Benjamin Fisch, vol. 169, 7–12.

(AJS) AMERICAN JOURNAL OF SURGERY

1964. The responsibility of the surgeon to surgery, by John R. Derrick, vol. 108, 670–72.

1965a. Objectives and principles in the training of the obstetrician-gynecologist, by Howard C. Taylor Jr., vol. 110, 35–43.

1965b. Touching all bases, by Leland S. McKittrick, vol. 109, 57–62.

1965c. Unnecessary surgery and technical competence, by Oliver Cope, vol. 110, 119–23.

1966. The triumvirate of medicine, by O. E. Grua, vol. 112, 623–26.

1967. The failure of surgeons as scientists, by Harvey R. Butcher Jr., vol. 113, 725–26.

1970. A look to the future of training in general surgery, by George Crile Jr., vol. 119, 221.

1971a. An improved rigid choledochoscope, by J. Manny Shore, Leon Morgenstern, and George Berci, vol. 122, 567–68.

1971b. The teaching of surgical judgment, by Robert M. Bartlett, vol. 121, 220–22.

1973. Extinction of the rotating internship, by Fikri H. Shabanah, vol. 125, 659–60.

1974a. Discussion, by George R. Dunlop, vol. 127, 467–68.

1974b. The passion and action of our time and surgical excellence, by James E. Bennett, vol. 128, 659–61.

1975a. Influence of choledochoscopy on the choice of surgical procedure, by Clarence J. Schein, vol. 130, 74–77.

1975b. Peritoneoscopy, by Walter D. Gaisford, vol. 130, 671–78.

1976a. A clinical teacher looks at surgical education, by Ralph D. Cressman, vol. 132, 140–43.

1976b. Discussion, by Lloyd M. Nyhus, vol. 132, 181.

1976c. Operative endoscopy in the management of biliary tract neoplasms, by Ronald K. Tompkins, James Johnson, F. Kristian Storm, and William P. Longmire, vol. 132, 174–82.

1977a. Doctor, is this operation necessary?, by Carl P. Schlicke, vol. 134, 3–12.

1977b. A hard look at colonoscopy, by Jerome S. Abrams, vol. 133, 111–15.

1977c. Operative choledochoscopy, by Paul F. Nora, George Berci, Richard A. Dorazio, Gerald Kirshenbaum, J. Manny Shore, Ronald K. Tompkins, and Stuart D. Wilson, vol. 133, 105–10.

1978. Colonoscopy and polypectomy, by Stewart M. Johnson, vol. 136, 313–16.

1979a. Endoscopic electrohemostasis of active upper gastrointestinal bleeding, by Walter D. Gaisford, vol. 137, 47–52.

1979b. Lower gastrointestinal bleeding with negative or inconclusive radiographic studies, by George J. Todd and Kenneth A. Forde, vol. 138, 627–28.

1979c. Operative and postoperative choledochofiberoscopy, by Norimasa Okabe, Keizo Kawai, Ohmi Kondo, Takashi Machida, Hiroshi Adachi, Tetsu Wtanuki, vol. 137, 816–20.

1980a. Choledochofiberoscopy in the postoperative management of intrahepatic stones, by Min-Huo Hwang, Jyh-Chung Yang, and Shuenn-An Lee, vol. 139, 860–64.

1980b. Choledochoscopy as a complementary procedure to operative cholangiography in biliary surgery, by Pacifico C. Yap, Mariano Atacador, Alexander G. Yap, and Richard G. Yap, vol. 140, 648–52.

1980c. Limited value of early endoscopy in the management of acute upper gastrointestinal bleeding, by David Y.Graham, vol. 140, 284–90.

1980d. A surgeon's view, by Darvan A. Moosman, vol. 140, 266–69.

1980e. Surgery of the alimentary tract, by George L. Jordan Jr., vol. 139, 3–9.

1980f. Surgical residency, by Ward O. Griffen Jr. vol. 140, 720–23.

1981a. Changing patterns of surgical training and practice, by William P. Longmire Jr., vol. 141, 632–37.

1981b. The scientist-surgeon, by Henry Buchwald, vol. 142, 245–46.

1982. Perceived needs for gastrointestinal endoscopic training in surgical residencies, by Martin H. Max and Hiram C. Polk Jr., vol. 143, 150–52.

1983a. General surgery, by Hilding H. Olson, vol. 146, 2–6.

1983b. Surgical gastroenterology, by Frank G. Moody, vol. 145, 2–4.

1984. Choledochoscopy in surgery for choledocholithiasis, by Jean Escat, Donald L. Glucksman, Christian Maigne, Gilles Fourtanier, Dominique Fournier, and Claude Vaislic, vol. 147, 670–71.

1985. Intraoperative biliary endoscopy (choledochoscopy) in California hospitals, by Alex G. Schulman and George Berci, vol. 149, 703–04.

1986a. Societal forces on surgery, by Ronald C. Elkins, vol. 152, 568–76.

1986b. What of the next 25 years? by James D. Hardy, vol. 151, 12–17.

1987a. A biliary endoscopy model, by George Berci and Alfred Cuschieri, vol. 153, 576–78.

1987b. Surgical handicraft, by Robert W. Barnes, vol. 153, 422–27.

1987c. What is a surgeon? by Joseph L. Kovarik, vol. 154, 563–77.

1988a. Gut reactions, by Ronald K. Tompkins, vol. 155, 2–5.

1988b. Nonoperative interventional therapy in gallstone-associated acute pancreatitis, by Joseph F. Patiño, vol. 155, 719.

1988c. Operative versus endoscopic gastrostomy, by Greg Stiegmann, John Goff, Charles VanWay, Lloyd Perino, Nathan Pearlman, and Lawrence Norton, vol. 155, 88–92.

1988d. Recollection, responsibilities, and rewards of a senior surgeon, by R. Edward Robins, vol. 155, 632–33.

1989a. Cholecystectomy, Charles K. McSherry, vol. 158, 174–78.

1989b. Cognitive nonsense, by Josef E. Fischer, vol. 157, 275.

1990a. Editorial comment, by Eddie J. Reddick, vol. 160, 488.

1990b. Editorial comment, by George Berci, by vol. 160, 488–89.

1990c. Electrocautery is superior to laser for laparoscopic cholecystectomy, by C. Randle Voyles, Albert L. Meena, Anthony B. Petro, Alexander J. Haick, and A. Michael Koury, vol. 160, 457.

1990d. Laparoscopic cholecystectomy, by Alfred Cushieri, George Berci, and Charles K. McSherry, vol. 159, 273.

1990e. Outpatient laparoscopic laser cholecystectomy, by Eddie Joe Reddick and Douglas Ole Olsen, vol. 160, 485–87.

1990f. A rural surgeon's perspective on general surgery, by Eugene H. Shively, vol. 159, 274–76.

1991a. The Baltimore experience with laparoscopic management of acute cholecystitis, by John L. Flowers, Robert W. Bailey, William A. Scovill, and Karl A. Zucker, vol. 161, 388–92.

1991b. Elective diagnostic laparoscopy, by Jonathan M. Sackier, George Berci, and Margaret Paz-Partlow, vol. 161, 326–31.

1991c. Emergency laparoscopy, by George Berci, Jonathan M. Sackier, and Margaret Paz-Partlow, vol. 161, 332–35.

1991d. The future of general surgery, by George L. Jordan, Jr, vol. 161, 194–202.

1991e. Graduate medical education, by George F. Sheldon, vol. 161, 294–99.

1991f. Granting of privileges for laparascopic general surgery, by Society of American Gastrointestinal Endoscopic Surgeons, vol. 161, 324–25.

1991g. Laparoscopic cholecystectomy, by Douglas O. Olsen, vol. 161, 339–44.

1991h. Laparoscopic cholecystectomy, by Jacques Perissat and Gary C. Vitale, vol. 161, 408.

1991i. March issue, vol. 161.

1991j. Minimal access general surgery, by Thomas L. Dent, Jeffrey L. Ponsky, and George Berci, vol. 161, 323.

1991k. A new technique of surgical treatment of chronic duodenal ulcer without laparotomy by videocoelioscopy, by Namir Katkhouda and Jean Mouiel, vol. 161, 361–64.

1991l. A practical approach to laparascopic cholecystectomy, by C. Randle Voyles, Anthony B. Petro, Albert L. Meena, Alexander J. Haick, and A. Michael Koury, vol. 161, 365–70.

1991m. Safe performance of difficult laparoscopic cholecystectomies, by Eddie Joe Reddick, Douglas Olson, Albert Spaw, David Baird, Horacio Asbun, Michael O'Reilly, Kerry Fischer, and William Saye, vol. 161, 377–81.

1991n. Traditional versus laparoscopic cholecystectomy, by Thomas R. Gadacz and Mark A. Talamini, vol. 161, 336–38.

1991o. Training, credentialling, and granting of clinical privileges for laparoscopic general surgery, by Thomas L. Dent, vol. 161, 399–403.

1992a. Incorporation of laparoscopy into a surgical endoscopy training program, by Bruce D. Schirmer, Stephen B. Edge, Janet Dix, and Anna D. Miller, vol. 163, 46–50.

1992b. Multipractice analysis of laparoscopic cholecystectomy in 1,983 patients, by Gerald M. Larson, Gary C. Vitale, Joseph Casey, John S. Evans, George Gilliam, Louis Heuser, George McGee, Mohan Rao, Michael J. Scherm, and C. Randle Voyles, vol. 163, 221–26.

1993a. Comparison of laparoscopic cholecystectomy with open cholecystectomy in a single center, by Lester F. Williams Jr., William C. Chapman, Roger A. Bonau, Edwin C. McGee Jr., Russell W. Boyd, and J. Kenneth Jacobs, vol. 165, 459–65.

1993b. Complications after laparoscopic cholecystecomy, by Harvey R. Bernard and Thomas W. Hartman, vol. 165, 533–35.

1993c. Exposure, dissection, and laser versus electrosurgery in laparoscopic cholecystectomy, by John G. Hunter, vol. 165, 492–96.

1993d. How American surgeons introduced radiology into U.S. medicine, by Ira M. Rutkow, vol. 165, 252–57.

1993e. Laparoscopic approach to common duct pathology, by Joseph B. Petelin, vol. 165, 487–91.

1993f. Laparoscopic cholecystectomy, by Jacques Perissat, vol. 165, 444–49.

1993g. Registry of laparoscopic cholecystectomy and new and evolving laparoscopic techniques, by John V. White, vol. 165, 536–40.

1993h. A review of 391 selected open cholecystectomies for comparisons with laparoscopic cholecystectomy, by Augusto Paulino-Netto, vol. 166, 71–73.

(AmS) AMERICAN SURGEON

1963. Choledochoscopy, by J. Manny Shore and Harvey N. Lippman, vol. 29, 731–36.

1972. Potentials of a new miniature optical system (endoscope) as a diagnostic aid, by Leon Morgenstern, J. Manny Shore, and George Berci, vol. 38, 312–13.

1981. Intraoperative choledochoscopy, by Thomas A. Broadie, Daniel K. Lowe, John L. Glover, Peter B. Yaw, and John E. Jesseph, vol. 47, 121–24.

1984. Intraoperative fiberoptic endoscopy, by William E. Strodel, Frederic E. Eckhauser, James A. Knol, Timothy T. Nostrant, and Thomas L. Dent, vol. 50, 340–44.

1986. Diagnostic laparotomy for abdominal trauma, by Gary C. Buck III, Martin L. Dalton, and William A. Neely, vol. 52, 41–43.

1989a. The impact of video endoscopy on surgical training, by Richard M. Satava and Stephen M. Gooden, vol. 55, 263–66.

1989b. Intraoperative and postoperative biliary endoscopy (choledochoscopy), by George Berci, Leon Morgenstern, and Margaret Paz-Partlow, vol. 55, 267–72.

(ARCSE) ANNALS OF THE ROYAL COLLEGE OF SURGEONS OF ENGLAND

1989. Choledochoscopy via the cystic duct, by Martin J. Dennis, Michael J. James, David Wherry, John Doran, and David L. Morris, vol. 71, 320–21.

1991. Arthroscopic and endoscopic skills, by David S. Barrett, Roger G. Green, and Stephen A. Copeland, vol. 73, 100–4.

(AnnS) ANNALS OF SURGERY

1963a. The credo of a surgeon, by Claude E. Welch, vol. 158, 740–46.

1963b. A definition of surgery, by Frank Gerbode, vol. 158, 775–77.

1967. The surgical residency revisited, by Oscar Creech, Jr., vol. 166, 303–11.

1968. The tempo of change, by Robert J. Coffey, vol. 167, 613–18.

1969. And gladly teach, by Rudolf J. Noer, vol. 169, 643–51.

1970. Operative biliary endoscopy, by J. Manny Shore and Ernest Shore, vol. 171, 269–78.

1971. The universality of surgery, by O. Theron Clagett, vol. 174, 325–32.

1973. Preoperative endoscopic cannulation of pancreatic and biliary ducts, by Michael Kozower, Richard A. Norton, Robert E. Paul Jr., Karim A. Fawaz, Harry H. Miller, Alan H. Robbins, Elihu M. Schimmel, Herman J. Sugarman, and Jaime G. Tomas, vol. 178, 197–99.

1976. Manpower goals in American surgery, by Francis D. Moore, vol. 184, 125–44.

1979. Surgical decision-making, by Ira M. Rutkow, Alan M. Gittelsohn, and George D. Zuidema, vol. 190, 409–19.

1980a. Intraoperative gastrointestinal endoscopy, by Talmadge A. Bowden Jr., Vendie H. Hooks III, and Arlie R. Mansberger Jr., vol. 191, 680–87.

1980b. Letter to the editor, by Watts R. Webb and Erle E. Peacock Jr., vol. 191, 388–89.

1981a. The current and future role of surgical physician assistants, by Henry B. Perry, Don E. Detmer, and Elinor L. Redmond, vol. 193, 132–37.

1981b. Experience with the flexible fiberoptic choledochoscope, by Joel J. Bauer, Barry A. Salky, Irwin M. Gelernt, and Isadore Kreel, vol. 194, 161–66.

1985. The contributions of infection control to a century of surgical progress, by J. Wesley Alexander, vol. 201, 423–28.

1986a. Percutaneous endoscopic gastrostomy, by Robert E. Miller, Bart A. Kummer, Howard I. Tiszenkel, and Donald P. Kotler, vol. 204, 543–45.

1986b. Postgraduate surgical flexible endoscopic education, by Charles B. Rodning, William J. Zingarelli, William R. Webb, and P. William Curreri, vol. 203, 272–74.

1986c. Postoperative flexible choledochoscopy for residual primary intrahepatic stones, by Tat K. Choi, Manson Fok, Martin J. R. Lee, Robert Lui, and John Wong, vol. 203, 260–65.

1991. Laparoscopic cholecystectomy, by Robert W. Bailey, Karl A. Zucker, John L. Flowers, William A. Scovill, Scott M. Graham, and Anthony L. Imbembo, vol. 214, 531–40.

(ArchS) Archives of Surgery

1971a. Adapt or perish, by Stanley O. Hoerr, vol. 103, 103–7.

1971b. Foreign medical graduates and surgery in the U.S., vol. 102, 532–33.

1971c. Women in surgery, by Carol C. Nadelson, vol. 102, 234–35.

1973a. Discussion, by Walter D. Gaisford, vol. 106, 462.

1973b. Discussion, by Alexander J. Walt, vol. 106, 454–55.

1973c. Gastroduodenal endoscopy, by Hubert M. Allen, Melvin A. Block, and Bernard M. Schuman, vol. 106, 450–55.

1973d. Gastroduodenal endoscopy, by Walter L. Peterson, vol. 107, 348.

1973e. Gastrointestinal polypectomy via the fiberendoscope, by Walter D. Gaisford, vol. 106, 458–62.

1974. Surgical manpower, by Robert A. Chase, Francis D. Moore, and Richard Warren, vol. 108, 637–53.

1976. The surgical assistant—that illogical regulation, by Basil R. Meyerowitz, vol. 111, 831.

1977. National surgical work patterns as a basis for residency training plans, by Francis D. Moore, Rita J. Nickerson, Theodore Colton, Seth Harvey, Richard H. Egdahl, William G. Babson, William V. McDermott, and W. Gerald Austen, vol. 112, 125–47.

1978a. Captain or engineer, by Ben Eiseman, vol. 113, 917–18.

1978b. Endoscopic electrocoagulation, by Nicholas A. Volpicelli, Jack D. McCarthy, John D. Bartlett, and William E. Badger, vol. 113, 483–86.

1978c. Surgeons in the United States, by Bernard S. Bloom, Walter W. Hauck Jr., Osler L. Peterson, Rita J. Nickerson, and Theodore Colton, vol. 113, 188–93.

1978d. What to do when physicians disagree, by Francis D. Moore, vol. 113, 1397–1400.

1979. Endosocopic papillotomy, by Murray G. Fischer and Charles K. McSherry, vol. 114, 991–92.

1982a. A decade of surgery in Canada, England and Wales, and the United States, by Eugene Vayda, William R. Mindell, and Ira M. Rutkow, vol. 117, 846–53.

1982b. Intraoperative biliary endoscopy, by Steven K. Kappes, Mark B. Adams, and Stuart D. Wilson, vol. 117, 603–7.

1983. The changing mission and status of surgery, 1780 to 1980, by Francis D. Moore, vol. 118, 1013–18.

1987. Fragmentation and specialization, by Claude H. Organ Jr., vol. 122, 639.

1989a. Seldom come by, by Clement A. Hiebert, vol. 124, 530–34.

1989b. The surgeon and biliary lithotripsy, by David L. Nahrwold, vol. 124, 769–80.

1989c. The surgeon, healer with work at hand, by John K. Stevenson, vol. 124, 1123–26.

1990a. Laparoscopic cholecystectomy, by Ronald K. Tompkins, vol. 125, 1245.

1990b. The surgical residency, by Walter J. Pories and Hazel M. Aslakson, vol. 125, 147–50.

1991a. The demise of general surgery, by Claude H. Organ Jr., vol. 126, 1335.

1991b. Laparoscopic hernioplasty, by Irving L. Lichtenstein, Alex G. Shulman, and Parvis K. Amid, vol. 126, 1449.

1991c. Laser and laparoscopic cholecystectomy, by David W. Easter and A.R. Moossa, vol. 126, 423.

1991d. Reflections on my surgical residency, by Michael E. Zenilman and Maurine A. Waterhouse, vol. 126, 1176–78.

1992a. Invited commentary, by David L. Nahrwold, vol. 127, 403.

1992b. Laparoscopic hernia repair, by Ira M. Rutkow, vol. 127, 1271.

1992c. Twelve hundred open cholecystectomies before the laparoscopic era, by Leon Morgenstern, Linda Wong, and George Berci, vol. 127, 400–3.

1994a. Can an academic department of surgery survive? by Jerry M. Shuck, vol. 129, 469–71.

1994b. Discussion, by Haile T. Debas, vol. 129, 912–13.

1994c. Discussion, by Stanley Klein, vol. 129, 913.

1994d. Discussion, Stephen N. Parks, vol. 129, 913.

1994e. Gallstone pancreatis, by Christian de Virgilio, Christopher Verbin, Lin Chang, Stuart Linder, Bruce E. Stabile, and Stanley Klein, vol. 129, 909–13.

1994f. Laparoscopic sonography, by Markus A. Röthlin, Rolf Schlumpf, and Felix Largindèr, vol. 129, 694–700.

(ATU) ALBANY TIMES UNION

1992a. Health panel endorses laparoscopic surgery, 17 September, B-13.

1992b. Murky future, by Sally Squires, 3 November, C-1.

1992c. Suit faults video surgeon in death, by Robert Whitaker, 2 April, A-1.

1992d. State moves to reduce errors in video surgeries, by Robert Whitaker, 14 June, A-1.

1992e. Video surgery questions hurt firm's stock, by Robert Whitaker, 19 June, B-13.

(BJOG) BRITISH JOURNAL OF OBSTETRICS AND GYNECOLOGY

1992a. Laparoscopic alternatives to laparotomy, by Ray Garry, vol. 99, 629–32.

1992b. Laparoscopic treatment of infiltrative rectosigmoid colon and rectovaginal septum endometriosis by the technique of videolaparoscopy and the CO_2 laser, by Camran Nezhat, Farr Nezhat, and Earl Pennington, vol. 99, 664–67.

1993. Can laparoscopic assisted hysterectomy safely replace abdominal hysterectomy? R. W. Hunter and A. J. McCartney, vol. 100, 932–34.

(BJS) BRITISH JOURNAL OF SURGERY

1986. Craft workshops in surgery, by P. G. Bevan, vol. 73, 1–2.

1987a. Operative choledoschoscopy via the cystic duct, by D. L. Morris, J. Harrison, T. Balfour, and D. C. Wherry, vol. 74, 613.

1987b. Surgical technique, by N. A. Matheson, vol. 74, 1190.

1991a. Role of intraoperative enteroscopy in obscure gastrointestinal bleeding of small bowel origin, by L. A. Desa, S. K. Ohiri, A. R. Hutton, H. Lee, and J. Spencer, vol. 78, 192–95.

1991b. Surgical training, by P. F. Jones, vol. 78, 1156–58.

1992. Laparoscopic *versus* open appendicectomy, by O. J. McAnena, O. Austin, P. R. O'Connell, W. P. Hederman, T. F. Gorey, and J. Fitzpatrick, vol. 79, 818–20.

1993a. Conventional *versus* laparoscopic surgery for acute appendicitis, by J. J. T. Tate, S. C. S. Chung, J. Dawson, H. T. Leong, A. Chan, W. Y. Lau, and A. K. C. Li, vol. 80, 761–64.

1993b. Laparoscopic herniorrhaphy, by I. G. Schraibman, vol. 80, 538.

1993c. Laparoscopic repair of perforated peptic ulcer, by C. K. Kum, J. R. Isaac, Y. Tekant, S. S. Ngoi, and P. M. Y. Goh. vol. 80, 535.

1994. Long-term results of highly selective vagotomy, by J. M. Wilkinson, K. B. Hosie, and A. G. Johnson, vol. 81, 1469–71.

(BJU) British Journal of Urology

1994a. Laparoscopic nephrectomy, by K. Kerbl, R. V. Clayman, E. M. McDougall, and L. R. Kavoussi, vol. 73, 231–36.
1994b. Laparoscopic urological surgery: 1994, by L. G. Gomella and D. M. Albala, vol. 74, 267–73.

(BMB) British Medical Bulletin

1986a. Biliary tract and pancreas, by D. L. Carr-Locke and P. B. Cotton, vol. 42, 257–64.
1986b. Colonoscopy, by Christopher B. Williams, vol. 42, 265–69.
1986c. Endoscopic instrumentation, by R. A. Miller, vol. 42, 223–25.
1986d. Introduction, by J. E. A. Wickham, vol. 42, 221–22.
1986e. Operative pelviscopy, by K. Semm, vol. 42, 284–95.

(CJS) Canadian Journal of Surgery

1983. The case against general surgery, by T. H. Brian Haig, vol. 26, 5–6.
1990. Laparoscopic cholecystectomy—fantastic? by N. Schmidt, vol. 33, 433–34.
1992. A technical-skills course for 1st-year residents in general surgery, by Alan G. Lossing, Elizabeth M. Hatswell, Thomas Gilas, Richard K. Reznick, and Lloyd C. Smith, vol. 35, 536–40.
1993a. The case of Canadian general surgeons, by R. H. Railton, William G. Tholl, and Claudia A. Sanmartin, vol. 36, 129–32.
1993b. Presidential address, 1992, by Frank W. Turner, vol. 36, 211–15.
1994a. Presidential address, 1993, by Marvin J. Wexler, vol. 37, 267–78.
1994b. The surgeon's ego, by Nelson S. Mitchell, Marilyn Kaplow, and Charles McDougall, vol. 37, 8–9.

(COG) Clinical Obstetrics and Gynecology

1976. Forward, by Clifford R. Wheeless Jr., vol. 19, 259–60.

(CurS) Current Surgery

1978. The surgeon-endoscopist, by C. Thomas Bombeck, vol. 35, 223–25.

(DCR) Diseases of the Colon and Rectum

1993a. Comparison between endoscopic laser and different surgical treatments for palliation of advanced rectal cancer, by W. Tacke, S. Paech, W. Kruis, H. Stuetzer, J. M. Mueller, D. J. Ziegenhagen, and E. Zehnter, vol. 36, 377–88.
1993b. Initial experience with laparoscopic appendectomy, by Kirk A. Ludwig, Richard P. Cattey, and Lyle G. Henry, vol. 36, 463–67.

(FS) Fertility and Sterility

1991. The role of laparoscopy in the treatment of endometriosis, by Andrew S. Cook and John A. Rock, vol. 55, 663–777.

(Gas) GASTROENTEROLOGY

1967a. Desirable characteristics of a clinical training program in gastroenterology, by the American Gastroenterological Association, vol. 53, 358–59.

1967b. Forward thrust, by Wade Volwiler, vol. 53, 367–70.

1969a. Analysis of academic training programs in gastroenterology for the 10-year period 1957 to 1967, by George A. Scheele and George Kitzes, vol. 57, 203–12.

1969b. NIH-supported training and research in gastroenterology, 1968, by Joseph B. Kirsner, vol. 57, 95–98.

1970. Training the gastroenterologist for academe, by R. M. Donaldson Jr., vol. 64, 338–39.

1975. Colonoscopy, by Bergein F. Overholt, vol. 68, 1308–20.

1976a. Complications of endoscopic retrograde cholangiopancreatography (ERCP), by M. K. Bilbao, C. T. Dotter, T. G. Lee, and R. M. Katon, vol. 70, 314–20.

1976b. Gastroenterology—1976, by Fred Kern Jr., vol. 71, 537–41.

1976c. Instruments for diagnosis, investigation, and treatment of digestive diseases, by Work Group X, vol. 69, 1151–60.

1976d. More on colonoscopy in inflammatory bowel disease, by Richard H. Marshak, vol. 70, 147.

1977. Guidelines for the training of gastroenterologists, by American Board of Internal Medicine, vol. 73, 382–85.

1978a. Editor's note, by John S. Fordtran, vol. 74, 1349.

1978b. Presidential address, by John A. Benson Jr., vol. 75, 353–56.

1978c. Overproduction of gastroenterologists? by David E. Langdon, vol. 74, 1348–49.

1979a. Clinical training in gastroenterology, by Fred Kern Jr., vol. 76, 1489–92.

1979b. Dear sir, by Michael O. Blackstone, vol. 77, 1163–64.

1979c. Endoscopy and gastroenterology, by Stanley H. Lorber, vol. 77, 1163.

1979d. On balance, by John S. Fordtran, vol. 76, 1492–93.

1979e. Reply to Dr. Fordtran, by Fred Kern Jr., vol. 76, 1493–44.

1979f. Rudolf Schindler, pioneer endoscopist, by Martin E. Gordon and Joseph B. Kirsner, vol. 77, 354–61.

1980a. Guidelines for subspecialty training in gastroenterology, by the American Gastroenterological Association, vol. 79, 955–57.

1980b. More on balance, by Fred Kern Jr., vol. 78, 174–75.

1981a. Manpower in gastroenterology, by Douglas W. McGill and John A. Benson Jr, vol. 80, 861–68.

1981b. Whither the American Gastroenterological Association? by Frank P. Brooks, vol. 81, 641–44.

1982. The AGA's quality control, by Malcolm P. Tyor, vol. 83, 953–56.

1985a. Changes in gastroenterology, 1960–1985, by Norton J. Greenberger, vol. 89, 933–38.

1985b. Lasers and cancer, by David Fleischer and Michael V. Sivak Jr., vol. 88, 605–6.

1986a. Endoscopic therapy of upper gastrointestinal bleeding in humans, by David Fleischer, vol. 90, 217–34.

1986b. Results of a membership poll, by Donald M. Switz. vol. 90, 482–85.

1987. The AGA rounds ninety and heads for one hundred, the presidential address, by Douglas B. McGill, vol. 93, 1155–8.

1989a. Fragmentation of bile duct stones by extracorporeal shock waves, by T. Sauerbruch, M. Stern, and Study Group for Shock-Wave Lithotripsy of Bile Duct Stones, vol. 96, 146–52.

1989b. Manpower in gastroenterology in the United States, by Irwin M. Modlin, Seymour M. Sabesin, William J. Snape Jr., and Walter Rubin, vol. 96, 956–62.

1992a. AGA governing board policy statement on training and education, by Ian L. Taylor, James Grendell, and Sidney Cohen, vol. 103, 1127–32.

1992b. American Gastroenterology Association, by Sidney Cohen, vol. 103, 1715–9.

1993a. Hospital credentialing standards for physicians who perform endoscopies, by American Gastroenterological Association, vol. 104, 1563–5.

1993b. Development and application of endoscopy, by Basil I. Hirschowitz, vol. 104, 337–42.

1993c. The specialization of gastroenterology in America, by Joseph B. Kirsner, vol. 104, 6–11.

1993d. The viability of the subspecialty of gastroenterology, by Walter J. Hogan, vol. 105, 1601–7.

(GCNA) Gastroenterology Clinics of North America

1991a. Biliary extracorporeal shock-wave lithotripsy, by Gabriel Garcia and Harvey S. Young, vol. 20, 201–8.

1991b. Interventional radiology in gallstone disease, by Brian Goodacre, Eric van Sonnenberg, Horacio D'Agnostino, and Robert Sanchez, vol. 20, 209–27.

1991c. Treatment of cholesterol gallstones with litholytic bile acids, by Gerald Salen, G. S. Tint, and Sarah Shefer, vol. 20, 171–82.

(Gut) GUT

1987. Report of a working party on the staffing of endoscopy units, vol. 28, 1682–5.

1990. Endoscopic demands in the '90s, by Brian Scott, vol. 31, 125–26.

(GynO) Gynecological Oncology

1993. Laparoscopy using the left upper quadrant as the primary trocar site, by Joel M. Childers, Peter R. Brzechffa, and Earl A. Surwit, vol. 50, 221–25.

(IJF) International Journal of Fertility

1992. Laparoscopy bashing, by Stephen L. Corson, vol. 37, 266–69.

(JAMA) Journal of the American Medical Association

1970a. Improved endoscopic diagnosis of gastroesophageal malignancy, by Seibi Kobayashi, Joao C. Prolla, Charles S. Winans, and Joseph B. Kirsner, vol. 212, 2086–9.

1970b. The Yale Affiliated Gastroenterology Program, by Robert S. Rosson and Howard M. Spiro, vol. 212, 1683–4.

1971. Colonofiberoscopy, by William I. Wolff and Hiromi Shinya, vol. 217, 1509–12.

1974a. Endoscopic electrocoagulation in upper gastrointestinal hemorrhage, by John P. Papp, vol. 230, 1172–3.

1974b. Flexible fiberoptic colonoscopy, by Gerald Marks, vol. 228, 1411–3.

1975a. Drugs and operations, by Jack W. Love, vol. 232, 37–38.

1975b. Endoscopic complications, by Stephen E. Silvis, Otto Nebel, Gerald Rogers, Choichi Sugawa, Paul Mandelstam, vol. 235, 928–30.

1975c. Numerator without denominators, by David H. Spodick, vol. 232, 35–36.

1976a. Colonoscopy, by Thomas D. Crowson, William F. Ferrante, and J. Byron Gathright Jr., vol. 236, 2651–2.

1976b. Postoperative choledochoscopy via the t-tube tract, by James P. Moss, Joseph G. Whelan Jr., Robert W. Powell, Thomas C. Dedman III, and William J. Oliver, vol. 236, 2781–2.

1976c. Surgeons in the United States, by Walter W. Hauck Jr., Bernard S. Bloom, C. Klim McPherson, Rita J. Nickerson, Theodore Colton, and Osler L. Peterson, vol. 236, 1864–71.

1977a. Endoscopic electrosurgical papillotomy and manometry in biliary tract disease, by Joseph E. Geenen, Walter J. Hogan, Robert D. Shaffer, Edward T. Stewart, Wylie J. Dodds, and Ronald C. Arndorfer, vol. 237, 2075–8.

1977b. Endoscopic recognition of early carcinoma in ulcerative colitis, by Robert H. Riddell, vol. 237, 2811.

1977c. Splenic rupture following colonoscopy, by A. J. Telmos and V. K. Mittal, vol. 237, 2718.

1977d. Too many surgeons? by Rudolf H. De Jong, vol. 237, 267–68.

1980a. Gastrointestinal hemorrhage, by John P. Cello and Ruedi F. Thoeni, vol. 243, 685–68.

1980b. Is general surgery a dying specialty? by Earl Belle Smith, vol. 243, 650–51.

1981a. Endoscopic laser surgery, by William A. Check, vol. 245, 1623–4.

1981b. Who should be doing gastrointestinal endoscopy? by Melvin Schapiro, vol. 245, 577.

1985. Endoscopic management of gastrointestinal tract hemorrhage, by Diagnostic and Therapeutic Technology Assessment (DATTA), vol. 253, 2732–3.

1988. Gastroenterology comes of age, by Joseph B. Kirsner, vol. 260, 244–46.

1989a. The future of general surgery, by American Medical Association, vol. 262, 3178–83.

1989b. Surgery, in the days of controversy, by George Crile Jr., vol. 262, 256–58.

1992. Surgery, by Claude H. Organ Jr., and William R. Fry, vol. 268, 413–14.

1994. General surgery, by Elsa R. Hirvela and Claude H. Organ Jr., vol. 271, 1674.

(JRM) JOURNAL OF REPRODUCTIVE MEDICINE

1976. Gynecologic endoscopy, by Jordan M. Phillips, vol. 16, 103–4.

1992a. Laparoscopic supracervical hysterectomy using a single-umbilical puncture (mini laparoscopy), by Marco A. Pelosi and Marco A. Pelosi III, vol. 37, 777–84.

1992b. Laparoscopy using a simplified open technique, a review of 585 cases by Nicola Perrone, vol. 37, 921–24.

1993a. Decreasing the degree of hypothermia during prolonged laparoscopic procedures, by Michael R. Seitzinger and Lenore S. Dudgeon, vol. 38, 511–13.

1993b. Laparoscopically assisted vaginal hysterectomy, by J. F. Daniell, Bryan R. Kurtz, Gordon McTavish, Larry D. Gurley, Robert A. Shearer, Jill F. Chambers, and Stephen M. Staggs, vol. 38, 537–42.

1993c. Laparoscopic hysterectomy with the Endo GIA 30 Stapler, by Chyi-Long Lee and Yung-Kuei Soong, vol. 38, 582–86.

(JU) JOURNAL OF UROLOGY

1991a. Laparoscopic nephrectomy, by Ralph V. Clayman, Louis R. Kavoussi, Nathaniel J. Soper, Stephen M. Dierks, Shimon Meretyk, Michael D. Darcy, Frederick D. Roemer, Edward D. Pingleton, Paul G. Thomson, and Stephenie R. Long, vol. 146, 278–82.

1991b. Urological laparoscopic surgery, by Howard N. Winfield, James F. Donovan, William A. See, Stefan A. Loening, and Richard D. Williams, vol. 146, 941–48.

(LANCET) LANCET

1985a. Endoscopy or radiology, by Enno Hentschel, vol. 1(8436), 1049–50.

1985b. Upper intestinal endoscopy, by M. L. Clark, vol. 1(8329), 629.

1987. The shadow-line in surgery, by Richard Hayward, vol. 1(8529), 375–76.

1989. Peroperative endoscopy in Peutz-Jeghers syndrome, by Andy Petroianu and Dulmar Garcia de Carvalho, vol. 2(8676), 1403.

1992. Colons and keyholes, vol. 340(8823), 824–25.

1993a. 'Keyhole' surgery with fatal complications, by Diana Brahams, vol. 341, 170.

1993b. Surgical innovation under scrutiny, vol. 342(8865), 187–88.

1993c. Whither (or withering) surgery?, vol. 341(8845), 597–98.

(NEJM) NEW ENGLAND JOURNAL OF MEDICINE

1965. Shuttuck Lecture, by H. Rocke Robertson, vol. 272, 1029–36.

1973a. An answer in search of a question, by Thomas C. King, vol. 289, 687–88.

1973b. Operative work loads in one hospital's general surgical residency program, by Edward F. X. Hughes, Eugene M. Lewit, and Elizabeth H. Rand, vol. 289, 660–66.

1973c. Polypectomy via the fiberoptic colonoscope, by William I. Wolff and Hiromi Shinya, vol. 288, 329–43.

1974. Chasing the dollar—a case report, by Jeffrey L. Ponskey and James F. King, vol. 291, 741–42.

1975. Endoscopic papillotomy for choledocholithiasis, by David S. Zimmon, David B. Falkenstein, and Richard E. Kessler, vol. 293, 1181–2.

1976a. Doctors who perform operations (first of two parts), by Rita J. Nickerson, Theodore Colton, Osler L. Peterson, Bernard S. Bloom, and Walter W. Hauck Jr., vol. 295, 921–26.

1976b. Doctors who perform operations (second of two parts), by Rita J. Nickerson, Theodore Colton, Osler L. Peterson, Bernard S. Bloom, and Walter W. Hauck Jr., vol. 295, 982–89.

1977a. In defense of endoscopy, by David S. Zimmon and David B. Falkenstein, vol. 297, 1405–6.

1977b. To the editor, by Henry J. Tumen, vol. 297, 673.

1977c. Endoscopy, by David B. Falkenstein and David S. Zimmon, vol. 297, 116.

1977d. Simple method for removal of gallstones after duodenoscopic sphincterotomy, by Lothar Witzel, Walter Häcki, and Fred Halter, vol. 296, 1536–7.

1978a. Research does not hinder clinical training in surgery, by Arnold E. Katz, vol. 299, 961.

1978b. Research hinders clinical training in surgery, by Susan Adelman, vol. 299, 102.

1979a. The visible vessel, by Robert H. Schapiro, vol. 300, 1438–9.

1979b. The visible vessel as an indicator of uncontrolled or recurrent gastrointestinal hemorrhage, by William J. Griffiths, David A. Neumann, and Jack D. Welsh, vol. 300, 1411–3.

1981a. Rhode Island, by Francis D. Moore, vol. 305, 1341–3.

1981b. To scope or not to scope, by Harold O. Conn, vol. 304, 967–69.

1981c. Routine early endoscopy in upper-gastrointestinal-tract bleeding, by Walter L. Peterson, Cora C. Barnett, Herbert J. Smith, Michael H. Allen, and Desmond B. Corbett, vol. 304, 925–29.

1981d. Surgeons and surgery in Rhode Island, 1970 and 1977, by Donald C. Williams, vol. 305, 1319–23.

1982a. To the editor, by Bernard S. Bloom, vol. 306, 873.

1982b. To the editor, by John F. Morrissey, vol. 306, 869.

1982c. Routine endoscopy in upper-gastrointestinal-tract bleeding, by M. J. S. Langman, M. W. Dronfield, and M. Atkinson, vol. 306, 869.

1992a. Endoscopic biliary drainage for severe acute cholangitis, by Edward C. S. Lai, Francis P. T. Mok, Eliza S. Y. Tan, Chung-Mau Lo, Sheung-Tat Fan, Kok-Tjang You, and John Wang, vol. 326, 1582–6.

1992b. Therapeutic gastrointestinal endoscopy, by Peter B. Cotton, vol. 326, 1626–8.

(NYT) NEW YORK TIMES

1992. When patient's life is price of learning new kind of surgery, by Lawrence K. Altman, 23 June, A-3.

(OG) OBSTETRICS AND GYNECOLOGY

1993. Electrical cutting device for laparoscopic removal of tissue from the abdominal cavity, by Rolf A. Steiner, Edward Wight, Yona Tadir, and Urs Haller, vol. 81, 471–74.

(OGS) Obstetrical and Gynecological Survey

1993. The role of laparoscopy in chronic pelvic pain, by Fred M. Howard, vol. 48, 357–87.

(SCNA) Surgical Clinics of North America

1982a. Colonoscopy, by Hiromi Shinya, Mark Cwern, and Robyn Karlstadt, vol. 62, 869–76.
1982b. Rates of surgery in the United States, by Ira M. Rutkow, vol. 62, 559–78.
1982c. The reliability and reproducibility of the surgical decision-making process, by Ira M. Rutkow, vol. 62, 721–35.
1982d. The Study on Surgical Services for the United States (SOSSUS) and its impact on American surgery, by George D. Zuidema, vol. 62, 603–11.
1982e. Surgical manpower, by Francis D. Moore, vol. 62, 579–602.
1989a. Establishing an endoscopy unit for surgical training, by Richard M. Satava, vol. 69, 1129–45.
1989b. Intraoperative and postoperative biliary endoscopy (choledochoscopy), by George Berci, vol. 69, 1275–86.
1989c. The surgeon as endoscopist, by Gerald Marks, vol. 69, 1123–8.
1992. Laser use in laparoscopic surgery, by John G. Hunter, vol. 72, 655–64.
1994a. Cholecystectomy, by J. Lawrence Munson and Laura E. Sanders, vol. 74, 741–54.
1994b. Historical perspectives of biliary tract injuries, by John W. Braasch, vol. 74, 731–40.
1994c. Is there a dilemma in adequately training surgeons in both open and laparoscopic biliary surgery? by Robert Dunham and Jonathan M. Sackier, vol. 74, 913–21.
1994d. Preface, by Richardo L. Rossi, vol. 74, xiii–xiv.
1994e. Technique of laparoscopic cholecystectomy, by Horacio J. Asbun and Ricardo L. Rossi, vol. 74, 755–75.
1994f. Techniques of laparoscopic cholecystectomy, by John G. Hunter, vol. 74, 777–80.

(SGO) Surgery, Gynecology, and Obstetrics

1971. Surgeon and anesthesiologist, by Judah Ebin, vol. 132, 887–88.
1973. The surgeon and fiberoptic endoscopy, by Thomas L. Dent, 137, 278.
1975. The surgical gastroenterologist, by Walter D. Gaisford, vol. 140, 86–87.
1977. The value of laparoscopy in general surgical problems, by Ira H. Friedman, Martin B. Grossman, and William I. Wolff, vol. 144, 906–8.
1982. One solution to the dilemma of endoscopic requirements for general surgical residents, by James R. Starling and John F. Morissey, vol. 155, 65–66.
1985. Television choledochoscopy, by George Berci, A. G. Shulman, L. Morgenstern, M. Paz-Partlow, A. Cushierei, and R. A. Wood, vol. 160, 176–77.
1990. Fiberoptic endoscopy of the gastrointestinal tract in surgical training, by James O. Myers, Jerry J. Ragland, and Louis A. Candelaria, vol. 170, 283–91.

1992. Surgical laparoscopic experience during the first year on a teaching service, by Robert E. Miller and Fred M. Kimmelstiel, vol. 175, 523–34.

1993. A brief historical perspective and a comparison of the current systems of surgical training in Great Britain, Germany and the United States of America, by John Klaus-Dieter and Irvin M. Modlin, vol. 177, 622–32.

(SURG) SURGERY

1962. The hepatic ductal system, by Clarence J. Schein, Wilhelm Z. Stern, and Harold G. Jacobson, vol. 51, 718–23.

1966. The surgeon among doctors, by Douglas Robb, vol. 60, 948–49.

1968a. The general surgeons and the curriculum, by James D. Hardy, vol. 64, 577–81.

1968b. The role of the surgical specialties in medical education, by J. Hartwell Harrison, Thomas B. Quigley, and Warren J. Taylor, vol. 64, 587–94.

1970. Medical education, by J. Englebert Dunphy, vol. 68, 408–9.

1972. Surgical residencies, by Francis D. Moore, vol. 72, 659–67.

1973a. The surgical residency, by Frank C. Spencer, Keith Reemtsma, and Paul A. Ebert, vol. 74, 791–93.

1973b. The young surgeon's dilemma, by John A. Drews, vol. 74, 634–35.

1974. Surgical anatomy, by John E. Skandalakis, Joseph S. Rowe Jr., and Stephen W. Gray, vol. 75, 148–49.

1976. Questionnaire on surgical manpower and residency training, by John H. Siegel, Hiram C. Polk Jr., and David B. Skinner, vol. 80, 277–82.

1977. Surgeons in the United States, by Bernard S. Bloom, Walter W. Hauck Jr., Osler L. Peterson, Rita J. Nickerson, and Theodore Colton, vol. 82, 635–42.

1978a. The fragile ecosystem of resident serfs, faculty yogis, and surgical commissars, by Alexander J. Walt, vol. 84, 295–300.

1978b. Surgical manpower and public policy, by Francis D. Moore, George D. Zuidema, and Walter F. Ballinger, vol. 83, 116–20.

1978c. Training and use of surgeon's assistants, by Henry L. Laws, Margaret K. Kirklin, Arnold G. Diethelm, Jaqueline Hall, and John W. Kirklin, vol. 83, 445–50.

1980a. Clinical performance versus in-training examinations as measures of surgical competence, by Harold L. Lazar, Edward C. DeLand, and Ronald K. Tompkins, vol. 87, 357–62.

1980b. Pitfalls in randomized surgical trials, by Willem van der Linden, vol. 87, 258–62.

1981a. Alice through the looking glass—anesthesiology for the surgeon, by Mark C. Rogers, vol. 90, 919–21.

1981b. Presidential address, by Robert J. Freeark, vol. 90, 565–75.

1981c. Surgical rates in the United States, by Ira M. Rutkow and George D. Zuidema, vol. 89, 151–62.

1983a. The creation of a surgical endoscopy training program, by Brian F. Smale, Howard A. Reber, Boyd E. Terry, and Donald Silver, vol. 94, 180–85.

1983b. University surgeons during rapid transition, by Douglas W. Wilmore, vol. 94, 121–25.

1985. Presidential address, by Lloyd M. Nyhus, vol. 98, 619–24.

1988. Presidential address, by Michael J. Zinner, vol. 104, 115–18.

1989. Presidential address, by Robert J. Baker, vol. 106, 581–88.

1990. The 'right stuff,' by Jon B. Morris and William J. Schirmer, vol. 108, 71–90.

Index